The EVERYTHING.
Glycemic Index Cookbook

Dear Reader,

This book is designed to broaden your recipe horizons when it comes to healthy eating. The research has been extensive and thorough. You will learn what veggies are loaded with carbohydrates and high on the Glycemic Index (GI) and which are low.

You'll learn how to mix the high GI and high carbohydrate foods with low to create a style of eating that both satisfies you and helps you control almost any condition based on diet. Whether you have diabetes, hypoglycemia, a heart condition, or are obese, you may find you are eating better because you are food-savvy.

When you need energy for strenuous activities, you can draw on your diet to provide it. When you are sitting at a desk and must stay alert, you can plan your diet around that activity, decreasing hunger pangs by snacking intelligently.

This book is all about intelligent consumption of a variety of foods for maximum health. Isn't that what we all want?

Here's to the delicious recipes that will make you feel wonderful and look terrific, too. Enjoy!

Nancy T. Maar

The EVERYTHING Series

Editorial

Publishing Director	Gary M. Krebs
Director of Product Development	Paula Munier
Associate Managing Editor	Laura M. Daly
Associate Copy Chief	Brett Palana-Shanahan
Acquisitions Editor	Kate Burgo
Development Editor	Rachel Engelson
Associate Production Editor	Casey Ebert

Production

Director of Manufacturing	Susan Beale
Associate Director of Production	Michelle Roy Kelly
Cover Design	Paul Beatrice
	Erick DaCosta
	Matt LeBlanc
Design and Layout	Colleen Cunningham
	Holly Curtis
	Sorae Lee
Series Cover Artist	Barry Littmann

THE
EVERYTHING®
GLYCEMIC INDEX
COOKBOOK

300 appetizing recipes to keep your weight down and energy up!

Nancy T. Maar, coauthor of
The Everything Gluten Free Cookbook,
with technical review by Barb Pearl, M.S., R.N., L.D.

Adams Media
Avon, Massachusetts

This book is dedicated to my mother, Patricia Walsh Toensmeier, whose fight on behalf of diabetics for good-tasting sugar-free candies and drinks was tireless. She would love this book!

An Everything® Series Book.
Everything® and everything.com® are registered trademarks of F+W Publications, Inc.

Published by Adams Media, an F+W Publications Company
57 Littlefield Street, Avon, MA 02322. U.S.A.
www.adamsmedia.com

ISBN: 1-59337-581-6
Printed in the United States of America.

J I H G F E D C B A

Library of Congress Cataloging-in-Publication Data
Maar, Nancy.
The everything glycemic index cookbook / Nancy T. Maar.
p.   cm.
Includes index.
ISBN 1-59337-581-6
1. Low-carbohydrate diet--Recipes. 2. Glycemic index. I. Title. II. Series.
RM237.73.M33 2006
641.5'6383--dc22
                                                2006004161

This publication is designed to provide accurate and authoritative information with regard to the subject matter covered. It is sold with the understanding that the publisher is not engaged in rendering legal, accounting, or other professional advice. If legal advice or other expert assistance is required, the services of a competent professional person should be sought.
—From a *Declaration of Principles* jointly adopted by a Committee of the American Bar Association and a Committee of Publishers and Associations

Many of the designations used by manufacturers and sellers to distinguish their products are claimed as trademarks. Where those designations appear in this book and Adams Media was aware of a trademark claim, the designations have been printed with initial capital letters.

This book is available at quantity discounts for bulk purchases.
For information, please call 1-800-872-5627.

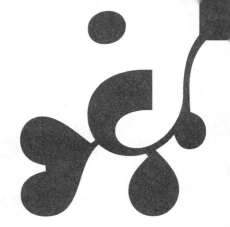

Contents

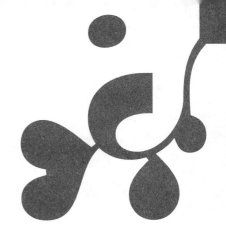

Acknowledgments

Many thanks go to editor Kate Burgo for her understanding.

I can't say enough good things or sufficiently express my gratitude to Ellen Stringer for her organizational prowess and diligence. She faithfully figured the stats and pre-edited the recipes, making sure that I didn't make any dangerous assumptions that would have left the reader wondering what I meant.

I must also thank my husband, Leonard Maar, for his years of encouraging me to write. He's been my biggest fan for many years.

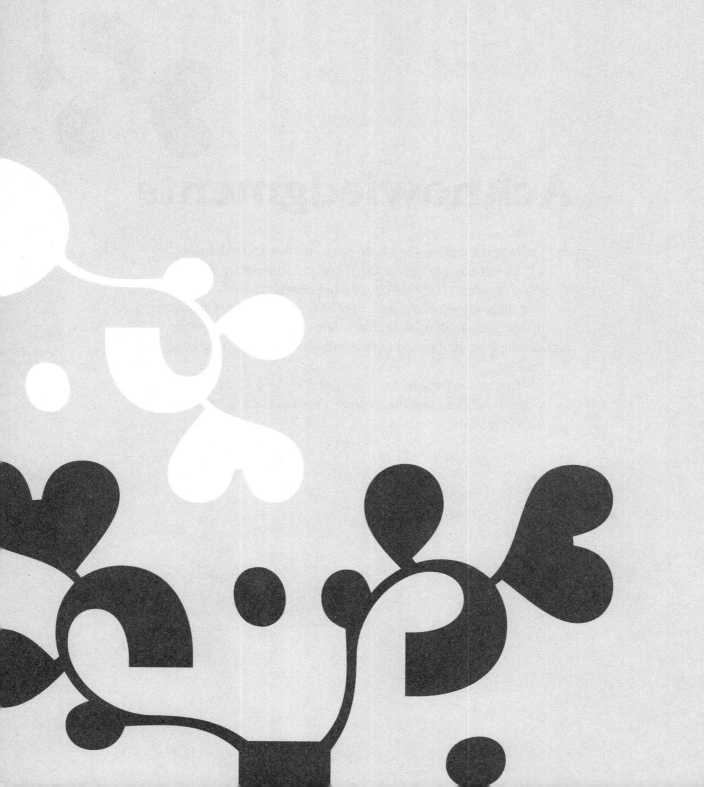

Introduction

The other night while fixing a dinner of baked fish, baby artichokes stuffed with garlic and cheese, and a big salad, I thought of how delicious this dinner would be. How healthy and satisfying! A dessert of fresh fruit made it both low calorie and filling.

When I began creating recipes for this cookbook, I had a special interest in the topic of controlling blood sugar by making dietary changes. My mother contracted type 2 diabetes in her early sixties, and my sister is hypoglycemic.

I often thought that my mother ate her way into diabetes. She'd skip a decent lunch or dinner and have two pieces of cake instead! Her body lied to her—giving her unhealthy cravings that exacerbated her heart condition.

As a result of my sister's condition, she has to be extremely careful not to overload her system with glucose or to allow her glucose level to drop excessively. The slow-release carbohydrates in the recipes listed in this book are perfectly suited to improve her health and energy.

Enjoying very good health and not wanting to contract either hypoglycemia or diabetes, I embraced this project with enthusiasm. As people get older, their metabolisms tend to slow. A meal that includes a fast-released carbohydrate coupled with a slow one will keep your blood sugar more level and maintain a comfortable level of energy for your body.

When you understand the Glycemic Index as your guide to meal planning, you will, with regular exercise, lose excess pounds, have loads of energy, and generally last longer at whatever you are doing. It works for me!

chapter 1
Understanding the Glycemic Index

The Glycemic Index (GI) is a tool to help you decide what to eat to help you achieve various goals, including increasing your energy and endurance, losing weight, and managing hypoglycemia and diabetes. This cookbook will teach you how to use the Glycemic Index to select satisfying foods that will provide you with healthy, long-lasting energy throughout the day.

What Is the Glycemic Index?

The Glycemic Index measures the speed at which your bloodstream absorbs the sugars in carbohydrates against a mean of 100, which equals the speed of glucose (pure sugar) absorption. In other words, the GI ranks carbohydrates based on their immediate effect on the pure sugar levels in the bloodstream. For more information about the GI and how to calculate the GI of specific foods, you may want to visit *www.diabetesnet.com*.

High Glycemic Index Carbohydrates

A carbohydrate that is ranked high on the Glycemic Index is a food that is digested quickly following consumption and causes a dramatic and immediate peak in glucose levels—giving the person eating a "sugar high," followed shortly thereafter by a sugar-induced low period. A classic example of this is the child who goes to school having consumed a breakfast of a sweet soft drink, frosted cereal, and a snack cake. This child is hyperactive for a short period of time, and then her energy level sinks radically. The child then feels tired, and she cannot pay attention to schoolwork during either the high or low states.

Low Glycemic Index Carbohydrates

A slow-release food is low on the Glycemic Index and crests at much lower levels, running slowly downward until it reaches the final stage of digestion in the large intestine. Thus, energy levels remain constant for a long period of time, and there are no rapid highs or precipitous lows. Healthy snacks can bump the energy level back to full strength when it starts to decline. An example of this is the school child warmed by a whole grain hot cereal, such as oatmeal, with milk and fruit. He will maintain a consistent energy level lasting until lunch.

Understanding the Numbers of the GI

People who have followed a low to moderate level GI diet claim that they feel more energetic, have lost weight more easily, and generally feel better. GI levels are included in the stats for each recipe in this book and, in general, are based on comparing measurements of the carbohydrate's effect on blood glucose levels with an equal carbohydrate amount of glucose alone. (So the Glycemic Index value of glucose by itself is 100.) The numeric breakdown of foods very low on the GI to high on the GI is:

Zero: There is no glucose in the food described.
Very Low: 10 to 35
Low: 36 to 55
Moderate: 56 to 69
High: 70 and up

Foods high on the Glycemic Index, that is, quick absorbers, force the pancreas to make a great deal of insulin, which is an essential hormone that regulates the sugars produced through digestion.

When high GI foods overload the pancreas, it produces an excess of insulin. When there's too much insulin, the energy created by the sugars is stored in the form of fat. Years of consuming large amounts of high sugary foods, coupled with weight gain, may "exhaust" the pancreas, causing less production of insulin and possibly leading to type 2 diabetes, (especially in individuals who are genetically predisposed to contracting that disease). Even if an individual does not contract diabetes, that person is likely to be obese and prone to heart disease.

Without an overabundance of sugars, insulin production is a fine and essential part of body function. It pumps the sugar (glucose) from carbohydrates into the bloodstream, which carries that energy to nourish the muscles and the brain. The muscles use glucose for the energy required to live—to walk, run, work, study, and play.

Getting Started: GI Guidelines

The GI gives you a guide to healthy eating. By choosing to eat low to moderate foods on the GI scale and exercising regularly, you can sustain your energy, prevent fat storage, help to avert heart disease, and keep brain function high, all without endangering your system. Before you get started whipping up low GI meals, there are some guidelines to help you learn the effects of certain foods on your glucose levels and choose wisely when planning meals.

Fats and Oils

Fats and oils modify the speed of absorption of high GI foods. For example, the fat in ice cream, to some extent, compensates for its sugar and lactose (milk sugar) content. Saturated fats such as coconut oil, lard, and butter can clog the walls of arteries, causing arteriosclerosis. Unsaturated and polyunsaturated fats, such as certain brands of margarine, olive oil, soy oil, and canola oil, are "heart healthy" and do not clog arteries.

Potatoes

Very high on the GI, potatoes are America's favorite source of carbohydrate. When fried or made into chips, potatoes are devastating to a healthy diet. A medium-sized baked potato, once or twice a week is fine, but if it's loaded with butter and/or sour cream, beware! You've gone from a potentially healthy vegetable to a high GI, high fat, and potentially artery-clogging combination.

Pasta

Pasta made from semolina is a good source of low-GI carbohydrates. Tomato sauce with many vegetables is excellent, and even a light, creamy sauce will reduce the GI.

Rice

Brown rice and basmati rice are excellent sources of slow absorption food, ranking moderate on the GI scale.

High-Fiber Vegetables

Especially fibrous vegetables, such as broccoli (including stems), cabbage, celery, peppers, and green beans, are very slow to digest and can slow down the digestion of foods higher on the GI (such as starches).

Breakfast Foods

Unfortunately, most breakfast foods are made with white flour, corn flour, or other finely ground, processed grains. Whole grains take longer to digest and hold up well in the energy department. Be careful to make sure that you are getting whole grains, however. While most people would assume oatmeal is healthy all-around, precooked and instant oatmeal are high on the GI. Old-fashioned oatmeal and especially imported brands of oatmeal (such as Irish and English oatmeal) are high in fiber and will digest slowly. This is also true of coarse cornmeal when used in cereal, muffins, and polenta.

Heart-Healthy Guidelines

As you read the recipes in this cookbook, you will notice a heart symbol paired with suggested substitutions for some of the recipes. This symbol indicates more heart-healthy alternative ingredients that you can use to lower the fat content and amount of calories in these recipes in order to maintain a diet suited to your own nutritional needs. These suggestions have been contributed by Barb Pearl, the technical reviewer of this text, and are aimed at readers who want to dine low on the GI while remaining conscious of caloric and fat intake.

chapter 2
Breakfast for the Active

Irish Oatmeal and Poached Fruit

This will keep the kids going for hours! It has the perfect combination of slow-release starch and get 'em going fruit. The nuts will stave off hunger, too!

Serves 4

Per Serving

Calories: 600
GI: Moderate
Carbohydrates: 61 g.
Protein: 32 g.
Fat: 36 g.

1 fresh peach, chopped
½ cup raisins
1 tart apple, cored and
 chopped
½ cup water
3 tablespoons honey
½ teaspoon salt
2 cups Irish or Scottish
 Oatmeal
1-½ cups nonfat milk
1-½ cups low-fat yogurt
1 cup toasted walnuts

1. In a saucepan, mix the peach, raisins, and apple with water, honey, and salt. Bring to a boil and remove from heat.

2. Mix the oatmeal and skim milk with the low-fat yogurt. Cook according to package directions.

3. Mix in the fruit and cook for another 2 to 3 minutes. Serve hot, sprinkled with the walnuts.

Substitute 1 tablespoon honey for the 3 tablespoons honey and use ½ cup of toasted walnuts instead of 1 cup.

Instant Oatmeal

Avoid instant oatmeal for breakfast, for cookies, and for making snacks. The oats in instant oatmeal are cut very thinly, and particle size is important to a low GI. The larger the particles, the lower the food is on the GI.

Sausage and Spicy Eggs

This is a very pretty and tasty dish that is not only a delicious breakfast, but is also good for lunch or a late supper. Be careful not to overly salt the dish— most sausage has quite a lot of salt in it, so taste first.

1. Cut the sausage in ¼ inch coins. Place in a heavy frying pan with the water and olive oil. Bring to a boil; then turn down the heat to simmer.

2. When the sausages are brown, remove them to a paper towel. Add the sweet red peppers and jalapeño pepper to the pan and sauté over medium heat for 5 minutes.

3. While the peppers sauté, beat the eggs and milk together vigorously. Add to the pan and gently fold over until puffed and moist.

4. Mix in the reserved sausage, garnish with parsley, and serve hot.

> *Substitute nonfat milk for 2% milk and vegetarian sausage for Italian sweet sausage.*

Serves 4

PER SERVING

Calories: 383
GI: Low
Carbohydrates: 8 g.
Protein: 35 g.
Fat: 23 g.

---

1 pound Italian sweet sausage
¼ cup water
1 tablespoon olive oil
2 sweet red peppers, roasted and chopped
1 jalapeño pepper, seeded and minced
8 eggs
¾ cup 2% milk
2 tablespoons fresh parsley for garnish

Dieter's Delight

When you dine low on the Glycemic Index and low in fat, you will lose weight. This is a power breakfast for one but can be doubled, tripled, or quadrupled easily.

1. Spray a pan with nonstick, butter-flavored spray.

2. Sauté the scallions, zucchini, and tomatoes until soft. Add egg whites and your favorite herbs, turning gently. Sprinkle with salt and pepper.

Serves 1

PER SERVING

Calories: 23
GI: Very Low
Carbohydrates: 2 g.
Protein: 4 g.
Fat: 0 g.

Nonstick, butter-flavored spray
2 scallions, chopped
½ cup fresh zucchini,
    chopped in thin strips
4 cherry tomatoes, cut in half
4 egg whites, well beaten
Fresh herbs of choice (parsley,
    basil, oregano, and
    thyme are a few)
Salt and pepper to taste

The Marathon Breakfast

This keeps you on the run all day! Runners tend to eat lightly or not at all before a race. Nuts are a very high-fiber food with some good fat. Both the fiber and the fat take quite awhile to digest without weighing you down!

1. Boil the oatmeal in enough orange juice to cover the oats.

2. When the oatmeal has absorbed the orange juice, add the nuts, raisins, banana, and honey or maple syrup.

Serves 1

PER SERVING

Calories: 672
GI: Moderate
Carbohydrates: 85 g.
Protein: 12 g.
Fat: 37 g.

½ cup 1-minute oats
Orange juice to cover oatmeal
    (about ¾ to 1 cup)
¼ cup your favorite nuts
    (not peanuts)
10 raisins
½ banana
2 tablespoons honey or
    maple syrup

 For this recipe, eliminate honey or maple syrup to cut back on sugar.

Chestnut Flour Pancakes with Nut Filling

Various flours are wonderful in pancakes, crepes, and regular baking. Unless you are on a gluten-free diet, they work best mixed with all-purpose flour.

1. Boil the chestnuts briefly so that you can peel off the thin membrane on the outside of the nut. Purée the chestnuts in the blender or food processor; set aside.

2. In a large bowl, mix dry ingredients. Using an electric mixer (or old-fashioned elbow-grease), slowly beat in eggs, milk, puréed chestnuts, honey, and butter.

3. Spray a griddle or large frying pan with nonstick spray; place on medium heat. Drop half ladlefuls of the batter onto the griddle. Turn when bubbles rise. Respray often.

4. Use syrup or any type of poached fruit to top pancakes.

Substitute 2 ounces heart-healthy margarine for butter.

Serves 6

PER SERVING (3 PANCAKES)

Calories: 165
GI: Moderate
Carbohydrates: 24 g.
Protein: 6 g.
Fat: 7 g.

½ cup canned chestnuts
1-½ cups all-purpose flour
½ teaspoon salt
2 teaspoons baking powder
½ teaspoon baking soda
2 eggs
1 cup nonfat milk
2 tablespoons honey
2 ounces butter, melted
½ teaspoon salt, or to taste
Nonstick spray

Banana Chocolate Pecan Pancakes

What a great brunch dish!
These are a rich and luxurious breakfast treat, yet low on the GI scale.

Serves 4

PER SERVING (PLAIN)

Calories: 200
GI: Low
Carbohydrates: 24 g.
Protein: 10 g.
Fat: 7 g.

2 1-ounce squares semisweet
    baker's chocolate
1 cup pecans
1 cup whole wheat flour
2 teaspoons baking powder
½ teaspoon salt
3 eggs, well beaten
¾ cup 2% milk
6 tablespoons honey, or to
    taste
1 teaspoon pure vanilla
    extract
Nonstick spray
2 bananas, peeled and sliced
    ¼ inch thick

1. Melt chocolate with 2 tablespoons water and set aside to cool slightly. Lightly toast the pecans and grind in a food processor or chop by hand.

2. In a large bowl, mix dry ingredients except the salt. Slowly beat in the eggs, milk, honey, vanilla, and salt and then chocolate.

3. Spray a griddle or frying pan with nonstick spray. Heat to medium-high. Drop the pancake batter, about 2 tablespoons per pancake, on the hot griddle. Cover with banana slices. Turn when bubbles form at the top of the cakes.

4. Serve hot with butter, marmalade, or chocolate syrup.

> ❤   *Substitute nonfat milk for 2% milk.*   ❤

Brown Rice and Spiced Peaches

This is an excellent cold weather breakfast. You can prepare the rice and peaches in advance, mixing in milk and honey as desired, and heat in your microwave.

1. Boil water. Cook rice in salted water until tender, following package directions.

2. In a separate saucepan, mix peaches, spices, lemon juice, and honey. Bring to a boil and set aside.

3. When ready to serve, mix the peaches and rice. Add warm milk and more honey if desired.

Serves 4

PER SERVING

Calories: 260
GI: Low
Carbohydrates: 60 g.
Protein: 153 g.
Fat: 1 g.

1-½ cups brown rice
3 cups water
1 teaspoon salt
2 cups fresh or frozen peaches, or canned peaches in water (no syrup) with ¾ cup natural juices
½ teaspoon cinnamon
¼ teaspoon nutmeg
Juice of ½ lemon
2 teaspoons honey

Brain Food Breakfast

This recipe is perfect for when you have a major presentation, the kids have tests, or any other stressful time. Remember: Carbohydrates fuel the brain!

Serves 1

PER SERVING

Calories: 491
GI: Moderate
Carbohydrates: 63 g.
Protein: 17 g.
Fat: 22 g.

*½ cup cooked regular
    oatmeal (not instant)*
½ banana
2 teaspoons honey
½ cup 2% milk
1 soft-boiled egg
1 slice whole grain toast
½ ounce butter

1. When the oatmeal is cooked, slice the banana into it, drizzle with honey, and add milk.

2. Placing the egg on a teaspoon, lower it into simmering water for 2-½ minutes. Run under cold water; peel off shell. Serve on buttered whole grain toast with oatmeal on the side.

 Substitute nonfat milk for 2% milk in this recipe, and replace butter with heart-healthy margarine.

Grilled Vegetable Omelet

Whenever you fire up your outdoor grill, throw on a few extra vegetables! Cut them in halves or skewer them in large chunks. Drizzle with some herbs and oil and put the extras in a plastic bag for future use.

1. Mix together olive oil, garlic, rosemary, and basil. Let rest for 2 hours to develop the flavors.

2. Skewer vegetables and paint with the olive oil mixture. Sprinkle with salt and pepper. Grill until crisp-tender and slightly softened.

3. Prepare a large frying pan with nonstick spray; place over medium heat. Whisk together eggs, milk, salt and pepper, and Parmesan cheese.

4. Pour the egg mixture into the pan. Arrange vegetables across the center of the omelet. When it just starts to set, flip unfilled sides over the center. Reduce heat to low, cover, and cook for another 4 to 5 minutes.

5. Serve with more cheese or, if you like, sautéed mushrooms. Garnish with extra herbs.

Serves 4

PER SERVING

Calories: 365
GI: Low
Carbohydrates: 15 g.
Protein: 21 g.
Fat: 25 g.

¼ cup extra-virgin olive oil
2 garlic cloves, chopped
1 tablespoon fresh rosemary, chopped
¼ cup fresh basil, chopped
1 medium zucchini, cut in ½-inch rounds
1 sweet red pepper, cored
1 large sweet onion, cut in chunks
8 eggs, well beaten
½ cup nonfat milk
Salt and pepper to taste
¼ cup freshly grated Parmesan cheese
Nonstick spray

Spinach and Gorgonzola Egg White Omelet

This is diet and comfort food. The two don't seem to go together, but try this! The quick and easy spinach filling is a frozen spinach soufflé.

Serves 2

PER SERVING

Calories: 463
GI: Low
Carbohydrates: 16 g.
Protein: 37 g.
Fat: 28 g.

1 frozen spinach soufflé, defrosted
8 egg whites, well beaten
⅛ teaspoon ground nutmeg
1 teaspoon lemon zest, finely grated
½ cup Gorgonzola cheese, crumbled
Salt and pepper to taste
Nonstick butter-flavored spray

1. Prepare a nonstick pan with butter-flavored cooking spray. Make sure the spinach soufflé is thoroughly defrosted.

2. Place the pan over medium-high heat. Pour in the beaten egg whites and sprinkle with nutmeg, lemon zest, and cheese. Spoon 1 cup of the spinach soufflé down the middle of the omelet. Reserve the rest for another use.

3. When the omelet starts to set, fold the outsides over the center. Cook until it reaches your desired level of firmness.

The Versatile Omelet

The fantastic thing about an omelet is that you can stuff it with all kinds of things. Various veggies, fruits, and cheeses and combinations thereof make exciting omelets. Try mixing some Cheddar cheese sauce and broccoli or some Brie and raspberries for your next omelet and enjoy the flavors!

The Stevedore Breakfast

This is a breakfast for one doing hard, physical labor. It'll keep you warm, give you energy, and ensure there will be no letdown for several hours. Add juice and a banana for an extra energy boost with this meal.

1. Whisk eggs and milk together. Add the minced jalapeño. Soak the bread in the egg mixture until it is saturated.

2. Prepare a large frying pan with nonstick spray. Heat to medium. Fry the toast until brown on each side, about 4 to 5 minutes per side. Serve with sausages, bacon, or ham and desired sauce.

> *In this recipe, you can substitute nonfat milk for 2% milk and use Canadian bacon or vegetarian sausage instead of sausage, bacon, or ham.*

Serves 1 big eater

**PER SERVING
(WITH BACON)**

Calories: 572
GI: Moderate-High
Carbohydrates: 48 g.
Protein: 41 g.
Fat: 26 g.

4 eggs, beaten
½ cup 2% milk
1 jalapeño, seeded and
    minced
3 slices whole grain bread, cut
    ½ inch thick
Chili sauce or ketchup
Sausages, ham, or bacon
    (optional)
Nonstick spray

The Hiker's Breakfast

Oat bran cakes are perfect for hikers, providing slow-release, long-term energy.
Your stomach won't go to war to digest them, and you'll have loads of energy
for the long haul. These oat bran griddlecakes do the trick!

Serves 2

PER SERVING

Calories: 338
GI: Moderate
Carbohydrates: 61 g.
Protein: 11 g.
Fat: 8 g.

½ cup oat bran
1 cup low-fat buttermilk
½ cup dried cranberries
2 eggs, beaten until light
2 teaspoons honey
½ teaspoon salt
½ cup all-purpose flour
1 teaspoon baking powder
½ teaspoon baking soda
Options: maple syrup, apple
*   butter, any mono or*
*   polyunsaturated spread*
Nonstick butter-flavored
*   spray*

1. In a large bowl, mix together the oat bran, buttermilk, and cranberries. Let rest for 10 to 15 minutes.

2. In the blender, mix the eggs, honey, and salt. Slowly add the rest of the dry ingredients; then mix with the oat bran mixture.

3. Using nonstick butter-flavored spray, prepare a griddle and heat to medium. Drop cakes on griddle and cook until bubbles form on top, about 1 minute. Turn and cook until brown. Serve with choice of toppings.

The Vanilla Smoothie Breakfast

This basic smoothie will become a favorite in your house! Simple and delicious, it will fill you up with wheat bran and provide calcium through the yogurt.

Place all ingredients in the blender and blend until the ice cubes are pulverized.

Serves 1

PER SERVING

Calories: 262
GI: Low
Carbohydrates: 11 g.
Protein: 4 g.
Fat: 4 g.

1 cup low-fat yogurt, plain
1 package sugar substitute
1 teaspoon pure vanilla
   extract
2 ice cubes
1 tablespoon wheat bran

Smoothie with Chocolate and Coffee

At last, a smoothie for grownups! Try this one the next time you are entertaining friends. Dutch process cocoa is less acidic unsweetened cocoa that is less bitter than natural unsweetened cocoa and blends easily with liquids.

When the coffee and cocoa are dissolved, blend all ingredients in the blender and serve.

Serves 2

PER SERVING

Calories: 196
GI: Low
Carbohydrates: 28 g.
Protein: 12 g.
Fat: 6 g.

2 tablespoons instant
   espresso, dissolved in 2
   tablespoons hot water
2 tablespoons Dutch process
   cocoa, dissolved in cold
   water
1 package sugar substitute,
   or to taste
½ cup oat bran
1-½ cups plain, low-fat yogurt
1 tablespoon anisette liqueur,
   optional
6 ice cubes

Smoothie with Kashi

*This smoothie has a rich, nutty flavor from the Kashi powder that
makes it stand out from other blended fruit drinks.*

Place all ingredients in the blender and blend until puréed and
lump-free.

Peach and Raspberry Smoothie

*The mixture of raspberries and peaches is the basis of classic Peach Melba—
a wonderful dessert. This smoothie is rich and always sure to please.*

Place all ingredients in the blender and purée until well blended.

Banana-Kiwi Smoothie

Kiwi fruit are delicious, inexpensive, and a bit exotic.
They happen to be wonderfully loaded with vitamins as well!

Place the banana, kiwi, lime juice, and orange juice in the blender and purée. Add the rest and blend until smooth. Serve chilled.

Serves 2

PER SERVING

Calories: 237
GI: Low
Carbohydrates: 65 g.
Protein: 10 g.
Fat: 1 g.

1 banana, peeled, cut in
  2-inch segments
4 kiwi fruit, peeled, cut in halves
Juice of 1 lime
1-½ cups orange juice
2 tablespoons oat bran or Kashi
4 ice cubes
Optional—4 drops hot sauce

The Smoothie for an Adult Brunch

This is a decadent smoothie with chocolate liqueur and
peppermint schnapps that is for grownups only!

Place all ingredients in the blender. Blend until there are no ice chunks. Serve in goblets or champagne flutes with a sprig of mint for garnish.

Serves 4

PER SERVING

Calories: 234
GI: Moderate
Carbohydrates: 30 g.
Protein: 7 g.
Fat: 3 g.

2 cups plain, low-fat yogurt
1 teaspoon pure vanilla
  extract
1 ounce peppermint
  schnapps
2 ounces chocolate-flavored
  liqueur
1 tablespoon honey
½ cup low-fat vanilla ice
  cream
4 ice cubes
4 sprigs mint for garnish

Smoked Fish and Eggs with Grilled Tomatoes

Serves 4

PER SERVING

Calories: 326
GI: Moderate
Carbohydrates: 3 g.
Protein: 26g.
Fat: 23 g.

4 scallions, chopped
Nonstick butter-flavored
    spray
8 eggs
½ cup 2% milk
½ pound smoked salmon or
    herring, chopped
4 ounces cream cheese,
    softened
Grilled or Broiled Red
    Tomatoes (see page 23)

The people of the British Isles love their kippered herring,
Nordic people love all smoked fish, and what would an Irish or Jewish
breakfast be without smoked salmon, also called lox? This recipe is
somewhere between a frittata and an omelet and incorporates
the wonderful flavor of smoked fish into a healthy breakfast.

1. Spray a large frying pan with nonstick spray and add scallions. Sauté the scallions over medium heat until soft, about 3 minutes.

2. Beat the eggs and milk together and stir them into the pan with the scallions. Set the heat on low.

3. Sprinkle the top with salmon or herring and dot with cream cheese. When just set, cut in wedges and serve with grilled red tomatoes.

Substitute nonfat milk for 2% milk and low-fat cream
cheese instead of regular cream cheese.

Tomatoes for Breakfast

It seems that all over the British Isles, Spain, and the Mediterranean, you get grilled or broiled tomatoes with meals, from breakfast to dinner. They are perfectly delicious and very nutritious. Americans should have them more often!

Grilled or Broiled Red Tomatoes

This is an excellent side dish to accompany eggs.
The tomatoes pick up the flavors of any herbs used with them,
and you can add butter, cheese, and spices to flavor
the tomatoes in a variety of ways.

1. Cut the tomato in half, from top to bottom. Use a melon baller to remove seeds. Sprinkle with oil and herbs, salt and pepper.

2. Nest the tomatoes individually in aluminum foil with the top open. Place open-end up on the grill, over indirect heat. Close lid and roast for 15 minutes at 375°F.

Serves 1

PER SERVING

Calories: 67
GI: Low
Carbohydrates: 6 g.
Protein: 1 g.
Fat: 5 g.

1 large red, ripe, and juicy tomato
1 teaspoon olive oil or butter
1 teaspoon of your favorite herbs (rosemary, parsley, thyme, or basil)
Salt and pepper to taste

Fried Green Tomatoes

Serves 4

PER SERVING

Calories: 596
GI: Low
Carbohydrates: 22 g.
Protein: 6 g.
Fat: 57 g.

½ cup cornmeal
½ cup all-purpose flour
1 teaspoon baking powder
Salt and pepper to taste
1 egg
¼ cup 2% milk
2 very large green tomatoes
2 cups canola oil

If you loved the movie Fried Green Tomatoes, *you'll treasure this recipe!*

1. Mix the dry ingredients together on a sheet of waxed paper. Whip the egg and milk in a small bowl.

2. Remove stem and core of the tomatoes and cut in ½ inch rounds. Place in the meal mixture; flip. Dip in the egg mixture and return to the meal mixture.

3. Heat the oil to 350°F in a deep frying pan. Fry tomatoes until brown and crisp. Drain on paper towels.

 Substitute nonfat milk for 2% milk and 1 cup canola oil for frying instead of 2 cups.

Corn Cakes Topped with Fried Green Tomatoes

*These corn cakes are a crispy and slightly sweet alternative to
traditional pancakes. Paired with fried green tomatoes,
these are a satisfying and unusual addition to the breakfast table!*

1. In a large bowl, whisk the dry ingredients into the milk. Stir in the eggs, corn, and spices.

2. Prepare a griddle with nonstick spray. Heat to medium.

3. Drop cakes on hot griddle and flatten with spoon before they rise. Cook about 4 minutes per side. Turn when bubbles start to form on uncooked side.

4. Serve topped with fried green tomatoes.

Canned Foods

Some canned foods make a wonderfully convenient addition to the pantry. Canned tomatoes, beans, corn, and pumpkin are excellent for many purposes and save hours of time.

Serves 4 (16-18 cakes)

PER SERVING

Calories: 187
GI: Moderate
Carbohydrates: 34 g.
Protein: 9 g.
Fat: 3 g.

½ cup nonfat milk or low-fat buttermilk
1 cup whole wheat or all-purpose flour
2 teaspoons baking powder
1 tablespoon brown sugar
2 eggs, well beaten
¾ cup corn (cooked, fresh, or canned)
¼ teaspoon nutmeg
Salt and freshly ground black pepper to taste
4 Fried Green Tomatoes (see page 24)
Nonstick spray

Baked Grapefruit with Honey and Chambord

This is a super simple starter that never fails to impress brunch guests!
The Chambord and honey bring out the sweetness in the warm grapefruit.

Serves 2

PER SERVING

Calories: 79
GI: Low
Carbohydrates: 19 g.
Protein: 1 g.
Fat: 0 g.

1 large juicy grapefruit
2 teaspoons honey
2 teaspoons Chambord
   (raspberry liqueur)

1. Preheat broiler to 400°F.

2. Cut the grapefruit in half. Loosen the sections with a grapefruit spoon or short paring knife.

3. Spread the honey over the grapefruit halves. Sprinkle with Chambord. Broil for 10 minutes, but be careful not to burn.

Baked Avocados with Shrimp and Spicy Mayonnaise

This is an elegant and delectable recipe that makes
an impressive addition to brunch.

Serves 4

PER SERVING

Calories: 298
GI: Low
Carbohydrates: 11 g.
Protein: 8 g.
Fat: 27 g.

½ cup light mayonnaise
1 clove garlic, minced
1 teaspoon mustard
1 hard-boiled egg, chopped
½ teaspoon tarragon vinegar
4 scallions, chopped
2 ripe avocados, cut in halves,
   pits removed
Juice of ½ lemon
8 large, raw shrimp, shelled
   and cleaned

1. Preheat oven to 350°F. Place the mayonnaise, garlic, mustard, egg, vinegar, and scallions in the food processor or blender and pulse until well blended.

2. Arrange the cut avocados on a baking pan. Sprinkle with lemon juice. Place shrimp in the depressions left by the pits. Cover liberally with blended sauce.

3. Bake for 20 minutes or until shrimp is pink. Serve hot!

chapter 3
Appetizers

Caponata Baked with Brie

*Caponata is a very basic Italian vegetable appetizer,
most frequently associated with Sicily. It can be served on bread,
crackers, or in a sandwich and is wonderful for entertaining.*

Serves 8

Per Serving

Calories: 232
GI: Moderate
Carbohydrates: 9 g.
Protein: 5 g.
Fat: 21 g.

*1 green pepper, cored,
    chopped*
1 zucchini, chopped
1 small eggplant, chopped
2 cloves garlic, chopped
1 sweet red onion, chopped
½ cup olive oil
2 tablespoons capers
*10 green olives, seeded,
    chopped*
*1 tablespoon sweet basil,
    dried*
1 teaspoon oregano, dried
Salt and pepper to taste
*2 tablespoons red wine
    vinegar*
6-inch round of Brie
*1 sheet frozen puff pastry,
    thawed*

1. Sauté the vegetables and garlic in the olive oil over medium heat for 10 minutes. Add the herbs, salt and pepper, and stir in red wine vinegar. Cook for another 5 minutes.

2. Preheat the oven to 350°F. Roll out the pastry. Spread Brie on the pastry and spoon vegetables over all.

3. Bake for 25 to 35 minutes, or until pastry is nice and brown. Cut into manageable, appetizer-sized wedges and serve warm or at room temperature.

Puff Pastry with Brie and Raspberries

*This recipe is similar to Caponata Baked with Brie
(see page 28) but easier and quicker.*

1. Preheat oven to 350°F.

2. Roll out pastry and spread it with jam. Stud with raspberries. Place the round of Brie in the center of the pastry and bring pastry up the sides of the Brie. Pinch pastry together to close.

3. Bake for 35 to 40 minutes; set aside for 10 minutes. Cut into wedges and serve warm or at room temperature.

Frozen Puff Pastry

Frozen puff pastry saves a great deal of time, and it makes an elegant presentation. You can also use layers of Greek phyllo dough, and if you are in a major bind, you can use piecrust! The thinner you roll the dough, the lower the GI value.

Serves 6

PER SERVING

Calories: 152
GI: Moderate
Carbohydrates: 17 g.
Protein: 1 g.
Fat: 9 g.

1 sheet frozen puff pastry, thawed
3 tablespoons seedless raspberry jam
1 cup fresh red raspberries, ½ cup reserved for garnish
6-inch round of ripe Brie
1 ounce Chambord (raspberry liqueur), optional

Ceviche—Fresh Seafood in Citrus

This is a classical South and Central American appetizer. The citrus actually "cooks" the seafood, and everything else is a flavor addition.

1. Rinse scallops and pat dry in a paper towel.

2. Mix all ingredients except the olive oil in a nonreactive bowl. Cover and refrigerate for 8 hours or overnight.

3. Just before serving, sprinkle with olive oil. Serve in large cocktail glasses.

Serves 4

PER SERVING

Calories: 159
GI: Very low
Carbohydrates: 4 g.
Protein: 18 g.
Fat: 11 g.

½ pound fresh raw shrimp, peeled and deveined
½ pound raw tiny bay scallops
2 scallions, minced
1 green chili, seeded and minced
Juice of 1 fresh lime
2 tablespoons orange juice
1 tablespoon chili sauce
2 tablespoons parsley or cilantro
Salt and pepper to taste
2 tablespoons olive oil

Stuffed Mushrooms (Crabmeat or Shrimp)

These can be made in advance and frozen. This is very good party fare, but be sure you make enough—they go quickly!

1. Mix together everything but the mushrooms.

2. At this point, you can stuff the mushrooms and refrigerate or freeze, or you can continue the recipe.

3. Set oven at 400°F. Place stuffed mushrooms on a baking sheet and bake for 15 to 20 minutes. Serve hot.

Buying Mushrooms

Buy only the whitest, crispest mushrooms. If you buy them from a grower, you'll see that they stay white and unblemished for at least three weeks. Old mushrooms are tan to brown with black/brown flecks.

Makes 12 individual stuffed mushrooms

PER SERVING

Calories: 103
GI: Low
Carbohydrates: 5 g.
Protein: 3 g.
Fat: 8 g.

¼ pound cooked shrimp or crabmeat (canned or, even better, fresh)
1 cup soft white bread crumbs
½ cup light mayonnaise
Juice of ½ lemon
1 teaspoon fresh dill weed, or 1 teaspoon dried
Salt and pepper to taste
12 mushrooms, 1 to 1-½ inches across, stems removed

Makes 12 individual stuffed mushrooms

Per Serving

Calories: 54
GI: Low
Carbohydrates: 2 g.
Protein: 3 g.
Fat: 4 g.

---

2 tablespoons olive oil
¼ pound ground sirloin (very lean)
2 shallots, minced
1 clove garlic, minced
Salt and pepper to taste
1 teaspoon red hot pepper sauce, or to taste
1 teaspoon fresh gingerroot, minced
1 egg
1 teaspoon Worcestershire or other steak sauce
12 mushrooms, 1-½ inches across, stems removed
6 teaspoons fine white bread crumbs
Nonstick spray

Stuffed Mushrooms (Spicy Beef)

These disappear rapidly at a party—people love them!
As in Stuffed Mushrooms (Crabmeat or Shrimp) (see page 31),
you can make them in advance and either refrigerate or freeze.

1. Set the oven at 400°F. Heat the oil and brown the sirloin, shallots, and garlic. Stir in the seasonings, egg, and Worcestershire sauce. Set aside while you clean and stem the mushrooms.

2. Set mushrooms on a baking sheet that you have prepared with non-stick spray. Stuff mushrooms. Sprinkle with bread crumbs.

3. Bake for 30 minutes, until tops are brown and mushrooms are sizzling.

Stuffed Mushrooms (with Bacon and Herbs)

This is a delicious appetizer at brunch!
You could also serve these on the side with eggs.

1. Set the oven at 350°F. Clean mushrooms and place on a baking sheet that you have prepared with a nonstick spray.

2. Sauté bacon, onion, and mushroom stems until the bacon is crisp. Stir in bread crumbs, nutmeg, parsley, and sage. Let cool slightly and mix in the egg.

3. Spoon mixture into mushrooms. Bake for 20 minutes or until lightly browned and very hot.

Substitute Canadian bacon or vegetarian bacon for regular bacon.

Makes 16 individual stuffed mushrooms

PER SERVING

Calories: 23
GI: Low
Carbohydrates: 3 g.
Protein: 1 g.
Fat: 1 g.

---

16 mushrooms, 1-½ inches in diameter, stems reserved
2 strips high-quality bacon, cut in small pieces
½ red onion, minced
Mushroom stems, chopped
2 slices whole wheat bread, toasted and crumbled
Pinch nutmeg
2 teaspoons fresh parsley, minced
2 teaspoons fresh sage, minced
1 egg
Nonstick spray

Baked Stuffed Clams

*Try to use fresh clams rather than canned in this dish. Once you do,
you'll never go back to canned! Cherrystone clams are hard-shell
quahogs and are generally 2-½ inches in diameter.*

**Serves 4,
2 half clams per person**

PER SERVING

Calories: 195
GI: Low
Carbohydrates: 11 g.
Protein: 13 g.
Fat: 11 g.

---

*4 fresh cherrystone clams,
well-scrubbed and
opened, meat removed
1 tablespoon lemon juice
2 slices whole grain wheat
bread, toasted and
crumbled
1 egg
1 tablespoon mayonnaise
½ teaspoon dried dill
2 tablespoons butter, melted
Salt and pepper to taste
2 tablespoons Parmesan
cheese*

1. Preheat the oven to 350°F. Place the clam shells on a baking sheet.

2. Place the clam meat and the rest of the ingredients in the food processor or blender and pulse until mixed, but not puréed.

3. Spoon the stuffing into the clam shells and bake for about 20 minutes. Serve at once.

> ❤ Substitute 2 tablespoons olive oil or
> heart-healthy margarine for butter and low-fat
> mayonnaise for regular mayonnaise. ❤

Follow Your Nose and Your Ears!

When buying any kind of seafood, ask to smell it first. A fresh salty aroma is fine; anything else is suspect—don't buy it! When selecting clams, make sure that they are tightly closed and make a sharp click when you tap them together.

Baked Oysters (ersatz Rockefeller)

*The easiest way to make this is to buy shucked oysters and
bake them in commercially available scallop shells or ramekins.*

1. Spray the shells or ramekins with nonstick spray.

2. Divide the oysters among the shells. Sprinkle with lemon juice. Spoon the creamed spinach over the oysters and grate a bit of nutmeg over the top. Sprinkle with Parmesan cheese.

3. Bake for about 20 minutes, until the oysters are very hot and the cheese topping is lightly browned.

Serves 6

PER SERVING

Calories: 159
GI: Moderate
Carbohydrates: 10 g.
Protein: 9 g.
Fat: 7 g.

*1-½ pints shucked oysters,
   drained
Juice of ½ lemon
10-ounce box frozen creamed
   spinach, drained
Light grating of nutmeg
4 teaspoons Parmesan cheese
Nonstick spray*

Stuffed Celery

*This unique take on stuffed celery is wonderful,
replacing peanut butter or cream cheese with luxurious, buttery Brie.*

1. Lay the celery pieces on a cool serving plate. Remove the skin from the Brie and mash it with a fork. Mix in the capers.

2. Stuff each piece of celery and garnish with toasted walnuts.

**Makes 12 pieces
stuffed celery**

PER SERVING

Calories: 66
GI: Low
Carbohydrates: 1 g.
Protein: 3 g.
Fat: 6 g.

*Wide ends of 6 celery stalks,
   cut in halves
5 ounces Brie cheese,
   softened
2 tablespoons capers
3 tablespoons chopped
   walnuts, toasted*

Clams Casino

*This is great with tiny littleneck clams, which are sweet and tasty.
Some are saltier than others; so between the combination of the clams
and bacon, do not add any salt at all.*

Serves 4

PER SERVING

Calories: 238
GI: Low
Carbohydrates: 11 g.
Protein: 11 g.
Fat: 17 g.

16 littleneck clams, opened,
    juices retained
4 tablespoons butter
1 small onion, finely minced
Juice of ½ fresh lemon
2 teaspoons fresh parsley,
    chopped
½ teaspoon dried oregano
½ cup roasted sweet red
    pepper, chopped finely
3 tablespoons fine white
    bread crumbs
3 slices bacon, cut in 1-inch
    pieces
Freshly ground black pepper
    to taste

1. Preheat oven to 400°F. Place the open clams on a baking pan.

2. In a saucepan over medium heat, add the butter, onion, lemon, herbs, and red pepper. Mix well when butter melts and sauté for about 4 minutes. Mix in bread crumbs and sprinkle with pepper. Moisten with reserved clam juice.

3. Divide the bread crumb mixture among the clams.

4. Put a piece of bacon on top of each stuffed clam. Bake for 12 minutes, or until the bacon is crisp and the clams are bubbling.

*Substitute Canadian bacon or vegetarian bacon
for regular bacon.*

Caviar and Cream Cheese Stuffed Endive

These stuffed endives are elegant and very simple to make.

1. Lay the endive leaves on a chilled plate.

2. In a small bowl, using a fork, mix the cream cheese, sour cream, and dill weed with the lemon juice.

3. Spoon the stuffing into the endive leaves and place a few bits of caviar on each. Serve chilled.

 Substitute low-fat cream cheese and low-fat sour cream for their regular counterparts.

Makes 12 hors d'oeuvres

PER SERVING

Calories: 27
GI: Zero
Carbohydrates: 0 g.
Protein: 1 g.
Fat: 2 g.

*12 biggest leaves from 4
   plump endives
4 tablespoons cream cheese,
   room temperature
2 tablespoons sour cream
2 teaspoons dill weed
1 teaspoon lemon juice
2 ounces salmon caviar*

Lollipop Lamb Chops

This is an expensive appetizer, but it's worth every penny for a special occasion. Citrus zest (grated rind) in recipes adds pungent flavor. The aromas of orange and lemon zest infuse everything from meats to veggies and dressings.

1. Blend everything but the chops in a mini food processor or blender.

2. Pour into a large dish and add lamb chops, turning to coat both sides.

3. Broil or grill lamb chops for 3 minutes per side.

Makes 14 lamb chops

PER SERVING

Calories: 268
GI: Zero
Carbohydrates: 0 g.
Protein: 34 g.
Fat: 13 g.

*4 cloves garlic
4 tablespoons parsley,
   minced
3 tablespoons rosemary
Rind of ½ lemon, grated
3 tablespoons Dijon-style
   mustard
2 tablespoons olive oil
Salt and pepper to taste
14 baby rib lamb chops, have
   butcher leave long bones
   on and trim them*

Deviled Eggs with Capers

*If deviled eggs aren't spicy, they aren't devilish enough!
This recipe can be adapted if you want less heat. Deviled eggs are easy to
make and transportable—great for a picnic or brunch!*

Makes 12 half eggs

PER SERVING

Calories: 69
GI: Low
Carbohydrates: 0 g.
Protein: 3 g.
Fat: 6 g.

*6 hard-boiled eggs, shelled
and cut in half*
½ cup low-fat mayonnaise
*1 teaspoon red hot pepper
sauce, such as Tabasco*
1 teaspoon celery salt
1 teaspoon onion
1 teaspoon garlic powder
*1 chili pepper, finely minced,
or to taste*
*2 tablespoons capers, extra
small*
*Garnish of paprika or
chopped chives*

1. Scoop out egg yolks and place in your food processor along with mayonnaise, seasonings, pepper, and capers. Blend until smooth and spoon into the hollows in the eggs.

2. Add the garnish of paprika or chives and chill, covered with aluminum foil tented above the egg yolk mixture.

Brine-Packed Capers

Capers are actually berries that have been pickled. You can get them packed in salt, but they are better when packed in brine. You can get larger ones or very, very small ones—the tiny ones are tastier.

Maryland Crab Cakes

You can use imitation crabmeat in this recipe, but it's better to use fresh.

1. Mix together all ingredients but the oil and form into cakes.

2. Heat the oil in the frying pan to 275°F. Fry the cakes until well browned on both sides. Serve with tartar sauce.

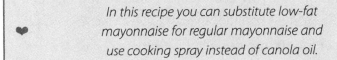

In this recipe you can substitute low-fat mayonnaise for regular mayonnaise and use cooking spray instead of canola oil.

Serves 4

PER SERVING

Calories: 494
GI: Low
Carbohydrates: 4 g.
Protein: 25 g.
Fat: 43 g.

1 pound lump crabmeat
¼ cup mayonnaise
¼ cup soft white bread crumbs
Juice of ½ lemon
1 egg
Salt and pepper to taste
2 tablespoons fresh parsley, chopped
½ cup canola oil for frying
Tartar sauce

Marinated Baby Artichoke Hearts

Here's where frozen artichoke hearts work perfectly!
They save you the time and energy of cutting out the choke and removing the leaves of fresh artichokes, and they taste delicious when marinated.

1. Thaw and cook the artichokes according to package directions. Drain and set aside.

2. Whisk the rest of the ingredients together in a bowl large enough to hold the artichokes. Add the warm artichokes and cover with dressing. Cover and marinate for 2 to 4 hours. Serve as antipasto.

Serves 4

PER SERVING

Calories: 142
GI: Very Low
Carbohydrates: 4 g.
Protein: 1 g.
Fat: 15 g.

2 9- to 10-ounce boxes frozen artichoke hearts
½ cup white wine vinegar
¼ cup olive oil
1 teaspoon Dijon-style mustard
½ teaspoon ground coriander seeds
Salt and freshly ground black pepper to taste

Caribbean Conch Fritters

Conch meat can be a bit hard to find, but you can order it on the Internet. These fritters are certainly worth the effort!

Serves 4, makes 8 fritters

PER SERVING

Calories: 383
GI: Low
Carbohydrates: 20 g.
Protein: 4 g.
Fat: 32 g.

1 pound fresh or frozen
   conch, finely chopped
½ cup onion, finely chopped
2 jalapeño peppers, seeded
   and minced
½ teaspoon curry powder
⅛ teaspoon nutmeg
½ teaspoon thyme leaves,
   dried
½ cup mayonnaise
1 egg, beaten
Salt and pepper to taste
1 cup dry white bread crumbs
Canola oil for frying fritters
Mango salsa (see page 90)

1. Mix all but the crumbs and oil in a bowl.

2. Form the fritters into egg shapes, roll in the bread crumbs, and refrigerate for 1 hour, covered.

3. Heat ½ inch oil in a frying pan to 350°F and fry fritters until golden brown all over, about 4 to 5 minutes.

4. Drain on paper towels and serve hot with mango salsa.

> ❤   *Substitute low-fat mayonnaise for regular mayonnaise.*   ❤

Frying Light

When you make fritters and other fried foods, it's important to use a very light oil, such as canola or safflower. Use regular olive oil for sautéing because it has lots of flavor. Extra-virgin olive oil is highly flavorful and expensive; it should be saved for salad dressings or to spritz on cooked veggies and pasta dishes.

Mini Codfish Cakes

*These are a wonderful appetizer,
served with tartar sauce or a great aioli.
(See page 238 for Aioli recipe.)*

1. Poach fish by submerging in boiling lemon juice and water until it flakes. Drain and cool.

2. Put the fish, egg, bread, dill, mayonnaise, salt, and pepper in the food processor or blender and pulse until coarsely mixed. Turn out on waxed paper.

3. Form into small cakes and sprinkle with bread crumbs.

4. Heat oil to 350°F and fry cakes until well browned. Serve hot or warm.

> *Substitute low-fat mayonnaise for regular mayonnaise.* ❤

Makes 12 small codfish cakes

PER SERVING

Calories: 303
GI: Low
Carbohydrates: 6 g.
Protein: 10 g.
Fat: 27 g.

1 pound boneless, skinless filet of cod
Juice of ½ lemon
½ cup water
1 egg
3 slices good white bread
1 teaspoon dill weed
½ cup mayonnaise
Salt and pepper to taste
½ cup fine white bread crumbs
½ inch light oil, such as canola, in frying pan

Baked Stuffed Artichokes

*These are worth a bit of effort. You can make them
in advance, then finish cooking just before serving.*

Serves 4

PER SERVING

Calories: 403
GI: Moderate
Carbohydrates: 54 g.
Protein: 15 g.
Fat: 16 g.

*2 large artichokes
2 tablespoons olive oil
2 cloves garlic, chopped
½ sweet onion, chopped
1 cup whole grain cracker
    crumbs, made in the food
    processor or blender
1 tablespoon lemon peel,
    minced
8 medium shrimp, peeled and
    deveined
4 tablespoons fresh parsley
4 quarts boiling water
Juice and rind of ½ lemon
½ teaspoon ground coriander
    seed
½ teaspoon freshly ground
    black pepper, or to taste
1 tablespoon Parmesan
    cheese*

1. Remove any tough or brown outside leaves from the artichokes. Using a sharp knife, cut off artichoke tops, about ½ inch down. Slam the artichokes against a countertop to loosen leaves. Cut in half, from top to stem, and set aside.

2. Heat the olive oil in a large frying pan over medium heat. Add the garlic and onion and sauté for 5 minutes, stirring. Add the cracker crumbs, lemon peel, shrimp, parsley, and pepper. Pulse in the food processor or blender.

3. Boil the artichokes with lemon and coriander for 18 minutes. Place the artichokes in a baking dish with ½ cup of water on the bottom. Pile with shrimp filling. Drizzle with a bit of the cooking water, sprinkle with Parmesan cheese, and bake for 25 minutes.

chapter 4
Entrée Salads for Lunch or Dinner

Blood Orange Salad with Shrimp and Baby Spinach

For an elegant supper or luncheon salad, this is a crowd pleaser.
The deep red flesh of the blood oranges contrasted with the saturated green of
spinach and the bright pink shrimp makes for a dramatic presentation!

1. Just before serving, place the spinach on individual serving plates.

2. Peel the oranges. Slice them crossways, about ¼ inch thick, picking out any seeds. Arrange on top of the spinach. Arrange the shrimp around the oranges.

3. Place the rest of the ingredients in the blender and purée until the dressing is a bright green. Pour over the salads. Serve chilled.

Fresh Spinach—Not Lettuce

Substitute fresh baby spinach for less nutritious iceberg lettuce. White or pale green lettuce can be used as accents but have less nutritional substance than such greens as spinach, escarole, chicory, and watercress.

Crabmeat Salad with Rice and Asian Spices

This seafood salad makes a wonderful main course for lunch or supper. Mild and delicious, Napa or Chinese cabbage keeps well in the refrigerator and adds an excellent crunch in salads.

In a large serving bowl, toss the cabbage, rice, and crabmeat. Mix together the rest of the ingredients for dressing and coat the contents of the bowl. Serve chilled.

Exploring Vinegar

Champagne vinegar is made from the same Champagne used for drinking. It is aged in oak barrels and because it is made from light, sparkling wine, it has a bright, crisp taste that is delicious in vinaigrettes.

Serves 4

PER SERVING

Calories: 471
GI: Moderate
Carbohydrates: 35 g.
Protein: 27 g.
Fat: 25 g.

2 cups Napa cabbage, shredded
2 cups cooked rice, brown or basmati
1 pound lump crabmeat, fresh (any kind)
1 cup low-fat mayonnaise
2 tablespoons champagne vinegar
2 tablespoons lemon juice
1 tablespoon sesame seed oil
¼ teaspoon Asian 5-spice powder
Salt and pepper to taste

Turkey and Apple Salad with Dried Cranberries

This is great for kids!
They will eat their veggies when presented as part of this salad.

Thickly slice the turkey and dice it. Toss all ingredients in a bowl with mayonnaise, salt, and pepper. Serve chilled on your favorite lettuce leaves.

> ❤ *You can make this recipe lower in calories*
> *by omitting the croutons and reducing the amount*
> *of mayonnaise to ¾ cup.* ❤

Chicken and Apple Salad

This is a marvelous way to use up leftover roast chicken. It has got everything
you need to feel good about your GI and your taste buds.

1. Place the rice, chicken, apple, and walnuts in a bowl.

2. Mix the curry powder, mayonnaise, and lime juice. Toss with the chicken mixture.

3. Place the lettuce leaves on plates and fill with salad. Sprinkle salad with salt and pepper and serve.

> ❤ *Substitute low-fat plain yogurt for the mayonnaise*
> *in this recipe to reduce the amount of calories.* ❤

Turkey Club Salad with Bacon, Lettuce, and Tomato

*This is a satisfying lunch salad, delicious and easy to make.
You can also put it on a bun and serve it as a sandwich.*

Thickly dice turkey breast. Fry bacon until crisp and crumble into large serving bowl. Mix all ingredients except the lettuce in the bowl. Serve over lettuce.

> For this recipe you can either omit
> the bacon or substitute it with vegetarian bacon
> or Canadian bacon.

Salad Dressings

Did you ever study the labels of commercial salad dressings? There are chemicals and preservatives in these dressings that you may not want to ingest. Save a nice clean bottle from olives. Make your own dressing and know that everything in it is healthy!

Serves 4

PER SERVING

Calories: 518
GI: Low
Carbohydrates: 14 g.
Protein: 40 g.
Fat: 34 g.

1 pound deli turkey breast
4 strips bacon
1 box cherry tomatoes, halved
1 head Boston lettuce, shredded
1 ripe avocado, peeled and diced
½ cup low-fat mayonnaise
½ cup of your favorite French dressing
2 cups lettuce, shredded

Portobello Mushroom Salad with Gorgonzola, Peppers, and Bacon

*The hot Gorgonzola cheese sets this salad apart
as an impressive main course or lunch.*

Serves 4

PER SERVING

Calories: 365
GI: Very Low
Carbohydrates: 12 g.
Protein: 11 g.
Fat: 31 g.

*2 large portobello
    mushrooms
½ cup French dressing (see
    page 92)
4 strips bacon, fried crisp
4 ounces Gorgonzola cheese,
    crumbled
½ cup low-fat mayonnaise
½ cup sweet red roasted
    peppers, chopped (from a
    jar is fine)
2 cups romaine lettuce,
    chopped*

1. Marinate mushrooms for 1 hour in the French dressing. Fry the bacon; set on paper towels and crumble.

2. On a hot grill or broiler, grill the mushrooms for 3 minutes per side. Cut them in strips.

3. While the mushrooms are cooking, heat the Gorgonzola cheese and mayonnaise in a small saucepan until the cheese melts.

4. Place the mushrooms on the bed of lettuce. Sprinkle with bacon. Drizzle with the cheese mixture and garnish with red roasted peppers.

---

*You can make this recipe lower in fat by substituting
your favorite low-fat cheese for the Gorgonzola and
by using vegetarian bacon or Canadian bacon.*

Mushroom Choices
There are many varieties of mushrooms now available. Brown mushrooms have a robust flavor. White button mushrooms are delicious in sauces, and the big ones work well when stuffed or grilled. Get wild mushrooms from a reputable mycologist. Never guess if a wild mushroom that you find in the woods is safe. It may be poisonous!

Grilled Shrimp Salad with Curry Dressing

*This is an excellent first course for an elegant dinner,
or with more shrimp, it makes a terrific summer supper.*

1. Skewer shrimp. Stir together the olive oil, curry powder, granulated sugar, lemon juice, Tabasco, and salt in a bowl. Place the shrimp in a large glass pan and cover with the dressing. Turn to coat.

2. Place the greens on serving plates. Grill the shrimp for about 60 seconds per side, or until they are pink.

3. Place the shrimp over the greens and garnish with the lemon wedges.

4. You can prepare more dressing for the greens, if desired.

Serves 4

PER SERVING

Calories: 245
GI: Low
Carbohydrates: 3 g.
Protein: 24 g.
Fat: 15 g.

*16 jumbo shrimp, peeled and
    deveined*
*4 wooden skewers, presoaked
    in water for 1 hour*
¼ cup olive oil
1 teaspoon curry powder
½ teaspoon granulated sugar
Juice of ½ lemon
2 to 4 drops Tabasco sauce
*1 teaspoon kosher salt, or to
    taste*
4 cups mixed spring greens
Lemon wedges

PER SERVING

Calories: 388
GI: Low
Carbohydrates: 13 g.
Protein: 3 g.
Fat: 39 g.

3 tablespoons sesame oil
½ cup olive oil
2 cloves garlic, minced
1 teaspoon fresh ginger,
    minced
2 teaspoons sherry vinegar
1 tablespoon soy sauce
2 to 3 cups Napa cabbage,
    shredded
¼ pound tuna steak per
    person (4 for this recipe)
1 red onion, cut in wedges
2 Japanese eggplants, cut
    lengthwise

Grilled Tuna Salad with
Asian Vegetables and Spicy Dressing

The fish is hot, the vegetables are spicy, and the greens are chilled!
This is an exotic salad that is deceptively easy to make.

1. In a bowl, whisk together the sesame oil, olive oil, garlic, ginger, sherry vinegar, and soy sauce and set aside.

2. Place the cabbage on serving plates. Paint the onion, eggplants, and tuna with the dressing.

3. Grill the vegetables and tuna for 3 to 4 minutes per side. Arrange the vegetables and fish over the cabbage. Drizzle with the rest of the dressing.

A Quick Meal

Tuna is a large fish in the Mackerel family that has a unique circulatory system that allows them to retain a higher body temperature than the cool waters they inhabit. This provides tuna with an extra burst of energy that allows them to reach short-distance swimming speeds of over 40 miles per hour!

Marinated Chicken and Brown Rice Salad with Water Chestnuts

Some salads, though not fattening, still are very filling. This is one!

1. Mix the red wine vinegar, mayonnaise, mustard, and celery salt together in a bowl. Spread 4 teaspoons of the mixture on the chicken breasts, being careful not to contaminate the dressing with a spoon that touched the chicken.

2. Combine the rest of the dressing with the cooked rice. Mix in the scallions, carrot, water chestnuts, salt, and pepper. Set aside.

3. Grill the chicken for about 4 to 5 minutes per side over high heat. Let rest for 5 minutes and slice.

4. Place the mixed greens on serving plates, mound the rice, and decorate with the warm chicken.

Serves 4

PER SERVING

Calories: 333
GI: Low
Carbohydrates: 33 g.
Protein: 5 g.
Fat: 21 g.

½ cup red wine vinegar
1 cup low-fat mayonnaise
1 teaspoon Dijon-style
    mustard
½ teaspoon celery salt
4 skinless and boneless
    chicken breasts, about
    4 ounces each
2 cups brown rice, cooked
4 scallions, chopped
1 carrot, julienne
1 8-ounce can water
    chestnuts, drained and
    sliced
Salt and pepper to taste
1 bag mixed greens, washed
    and ready to use

Wheat Berry Salad

Highly nutritious and full of vitamins and fiber,
this salad is ideal for breakfast or as a side. Wheat berries are
whole kernels of wheat that have a hearty, nutlike flavor.

4 cups water
1 teaspoon kosher salt
1 cup wheat berries
1 cup French dressing (see page 92)
2 cups jicama (Mexican turnip), peeled and diced
1 green apple, peeled, cored, and diced
½ pound small red grapes, seedless
Freshly ground black pepper to taste
2 cups leaves of mixed baby greens (from a prewashed bag is fine)

1. Bring the water to a boil. Add salt and wheat berries.

2. Cook the wheat berries until crisp/tender, following package direction.

3. Place cooked wheat berries in a large serving bowl. While still warm, toss with the French dressing. Add jicama, apple, and grapes. Toss and chill. Place mixture on plates over mixed baby greens. Add pepper to taste.

The Homely Legume

Jicama, also known as a Mexican turnip, is a lumpy root vegetable with a unique and versatile taste. The jicama's peel is inedible, but like a potato, it can be fried, baked, boiled, steamed, or mashed. The jicama can also be eaten raw. Try it as a vehicle for guacamole or use its mild flavor and crunchy texture in fruit salad.

Prosciutto and Jarlsberg Cheese Salad

Prosciutto is a sweet and pungent ham that is made in Italy and not smoked.
It's sugar and salt cured and then dried for a wonderful flavor.
Because it can be quite expensive, you can substitute it with country ham.

1. Toast the macadamia nuts in a toaster oven or in the oven. When toasted, chop nuts and set aside.

2. Arrange the lettuce on two chilled serving plates. Decoratively arrange the cheese and prosciutto over the greens. Sprinkle with pineapple and macadamia nuts.

3. Make a simple dressing by stirring together the olive oil, lemon juice, honey, mustard, salt, and pepper. Drizzle over the salad and serve.

> ♥ *You can reduce the amount of macadamia nuts and cheese in this recipe to lower the calories and fat.* ♥

A Chilly Nicety

When salads are to be served well chilled, the platter or dishes should be cold, too. Have you ever had a nice cold salad served on a plate just out of the restaurant's dishwasher? If you stick the platter or salad dishes in the freezer for just a few minutes, you'll find that your salads will taste better!

Serves 2

PER SERVING

Calories: 614
GI: Very Low
Carbohydrates: 19 g.
Protein: 24 g.
Fat: 53 g.

1-½ cups shredded romaine lettuce
2 ounces of thick-cut deli Jarlsberg cheese
¼ pound prosciutto, thin cut, shredded
½ cup fresh or drained, canned pineapple chunks
½ cup macadamia nuts
¼ cup olive oil
Juice of ½ lemon
1 teaspoon honey
1 teaspoon dark brown mustard
Salt and pepper to taste

Fig and Parmesan Curl Salad

*This mixture may sound a bit different, and it is!
In addition to being unique, it is also very delicious!*

PER SERVING

Calories: 284
GI: Low
Carbohydrates: 30 g.
Protein: 11 g.
Fat: 16 g.

---

*4 fresh figs, cut in halves or
4 dried figs, plumped in
1 cup boiling water and
soaked for ½ hour*
*2 cups fresh baby spinach,
stems removed*
¼ cup olive oil
Juice of ½ lemon
*2 tablespoons balsamic
vinegar*
1 teaspoon honey
*1 teaspoon dark brown
mustard*
Salt and pepper to taste
*4 large curls of Parmesan
cheese*

1. When the figs (if dried) are softened, prepare the spinach and arrange on serving dishes.

2. Whisk the olive oil, lemon juice, balsamic vinegar, honey, mustard, salt, and pepper together. Make Parmesan curls with a vegetable peeler and drizzle with dressing.

A Hidden Gem

Figs are a wonderfully nutritious food. Not only are they high in fiber and minerals, they also add tons of flavor to any recipe. Some cultures even claim that figs have medicinal value and healing potential.

Lentil Salad

This is a salad with a burst of protein from lentils.
Serve as a side or as a main lunch course.

1. Cover the lentils with water and add onion and wine vinegar. Bring to a boil, lower heat, and simmer until soft. Sprinkle with salt.

2. Toss with diced carrot and chopped celery and arrange tomatoes around mound of lentils. Sprinkle with French dressing and serve warm or at room temperature.

Serves 4

PER SERVING

Calories: 287
GI: Very Low
Carbohydrates: 25 g.
Protein: 7 g.
Fat: 20 g.

1-pound bag lentils (green, yellow, or red)
1 medium onion, chopped
½ cup wine vinegar
Salt
1 diced carrot
2 stalks celery, chopped
2 medium tomatoes, sliced
1 cup French dressing (see page 92)

Taco Salad

This is a great way to get kids to eat veggies!

1. Arrange the taco chips on serving plates. Sprinkle with cheese and place under broiler until the cheese melts.

2. Top taco chips with spinach, peppers, and onion. Serve with salsa and sour cream on the side.

> *Substitute low-fat sour cream for regular sour cream.*

Serves 4

PER SERVING

Calories: 489
GI: Low
Carbohydrates: 32 g.
Protein: 20 g.
Fat: 31 g.

16 taco chips
1 cup grated Cheddar or Monterey Jack cheese
1 bag baby spinach, shredded
2 sweet red roasted peppers, chopped
1 sweet onion, chopped
1 cup of your favorite salsa
½ cup sour cream

Meaty Spinach Salad with Eggs, Mushrooms, and Bacon

The meaty part of this salad is the portobello mushrooms and bacon.
The greens can be fresh or wilted, depending on your preference.

Serves 2

PER SERVING

Calories: 349
GI: Low
Carbohydrates: 7 g.
Protein: 13 g.
Fat: 27 g.

1 bag baby spinach, long
    stems removed
4 slices bacon
6-inch portobello mushroom
2 hard-boiled eggs, peeled
    and sliced
2 tablespoons Italian dressing
    (see page 92)

1. Arrange the spinach on two large dinner plates. Grill portobello mushroom and slice.

2. Fry bacon until crisp, drain off excess fat, and crumble. Decoratively arrange the bacon, mushroom slices, and egg.

3. Drizzle with Italian dressing and serve.

4. If you want wilted spinach, drop in boiling water for 1 minute. Drain and proceed as above.

> *Substitute vegetarian bacon or Canadian bacon*
> *for regular bacon in this recipe.*

Baby Vegetable Salad

Use the tiniest vegetables available for this salad.
Garnish with spicy prosciutto and sweet fennel.

1. Heat the olive oil over medium-low flame and sauté the garlic, onions, haricots verts, fennel, mushrooms, and carrots until the haricots verts and carrots are crisp-tender.

2. Stir in the champagne vinegar, basil, and parsley. Sprinkle with salt and pepper to taste.

3. When the vegetables are at room temperature, arrange the watercress and lettuce on serving plates and spoon on the veggies. Add tomatoes. Sprinkle with the ham and serve.

Serves 4

PER SERVING

Calories: 346
GI: Low
Carbohydrates: 18 g.
Protein: 19 g.
Fat: 20 g.

¼ cup olive oil
2 cloves garlic, minced
12 tiny fresh white onions
1 pound tiny haricots verts
    (baby green beans)
1 bulb fennel, rimmed of any
    brown and sliced thinly
5 ounces small white button
    mushrooms
8 baby carrots
¼ cup champagne vinegar
¼ cup fresh basil, shredded
¼ cup fresh parsley, shredded
Salt and pepper to taste
½ cup stemmed, loosely
    packed watercress
1 head Boston lettuce,
    shredded
½ pound currant or grape
    tomatoes
½ pound Black Forest ham,
    chopped

Poached Salmon Salad with Hard-Boiled Eggs

PER SERVING

Calories: 480
GI: Low
Carbohydrates: 7 g.
Protein: 36 g.
Fat: 33 g.

1-⅓ pounds salmon filet, skin and bones removed
½ cup cold water
¼ cup dry white wine
Juice of ½ lemon
1 tablespoon juniper berries, bruised with a mortar and pestle
4 hard-boiled eggs, peeled
1 cup low-fat mayonnaise
¼ cup stemmed, loosely packed fresh parsley
2 sprigs fresh dill weed, or 2 teaspoons dried
Zest and juice of ½ lemon
4 drops of Tabasco sauce, or to taste
Watercress or lettuce for arrangement on platter
Garnish of capers

This is marvelous for summer because you can poach the salmon the night before, chill it until ready to serve, and have a wonderful cold entrée. Adjust the amount of salmon to the number of guests invited, adding ¼ to ⅓ pound per person and an extra egg per person.

1. Place the salmon in a pan that will hold it without curling the end. Add the water, wine, lemon juice, and juniper berries. Over medium-low heat, poach the fish until it flakes, about 12 minutes depending on thickness. Do not turn. Drain and cool; refrigerate until just before serving.

2. In cold water to cover, bring the eggs to a boil and simmer for 10 minutes. Place under cold running water, crack, and peel. Slice just before serving.

3. Put the mayonnaise, parsley, dill, lemon zest and juice, and Tabasco in the blender. Puree until very smooth.

4. Arrange the salmon on a serving platter. Surround with watercress or lettuce and eggs. Dot with capers and serve green mayonnaise on the side.

Corn and Pepper Salad with Ham

When corn is in season, it's a great time to make a delicious corn salad. The addition of red and green peppers and ham to traditional corn salad makes this a perfect entrée for lunch.

1. In a small bowl, make the dressing by mixing the mayonnaise, cider vinegar, jalapeños, salt, and pepper. Set aside.

2. Mix the vegetables, ham, and chopped apple together. Toss gently with dressing and serve.

Grilled Corn

To cook corn on the cob, you can steam it, microwave it, boil it, or grill it. To grill, soak the ears in cold water before grilling (leaving the husks on). Then place the corn on a hot grill and close the lid. Turn the ears every 5 minutes until the husks are charred, then remove from the heat, husk, and serve!

Serves 4

PER SERVING

Calories: 438
GI: Low
Carbohydrates: 36 g.
Protein: 19 g.
Fat: 24 g.

---

1 cup low-fat mayonnaise
¼ cup cider vinegar
2 jalapeño peppers, seeded and minced
Salt and pepper to taste
4 ears cooked corn, cut from the cob
1 sweet red pepper, cored and chopped
1 green bell pepper, cored and chopped
½ pound country ham, cut in cubes
12 scallions, chopped
1 tart apple, cored and chopped

Filet Mignon and Red Onion Salad

There are few things that taste better cold than filet mignon!
Use a light salad dressing as both marinade and dressing.

Serves 4

PER SERVING

Calories: 501
GI: Very Low
Carbohydrates: 6 g.
Protein: 41 g.
Fat: 34 g.

1-¼ pounds well-trimmed
whole filet mignon
Salt and pepper to taste
½ cup French dressing (see
page 92)
1 red onion, thinly sliced
2 tablespoons capers
16 black olives, pitted and
sliced
Bed of romaine lettuce,
chopped

1. Preheat oven to 400°F. Place the filet mignon on a baking pan. Sprinkle it with salt and pepper. Roast for 15 minutes. Rest the meat for 10 minutes before carving.

2. Slice the filet mignon and place in a bowl with the French dressing, onion, capers, and olives. Toss gently to coat.

3. Spread the lettuce on a serving platter. Arrange the filet mignon, onion, olives, and capers over the top. Serve at room temperature or chilled.

Know Your Beef

Filet mignon is French for "small and boneless meat." This cut is the small part of a beef tenderloin and is considered the most delectable cut of beef because of its melt-in-your-mouth texture. Save yourself some money by preparing this at home instead of dining out!

Italian Seafood Salad

This salad gives you a great deal of latitude for using what is freshest in the market. This recipe is a starting place. You can substitute lobster for shrimp or use any kind of crabmeat. You can add other fresh herbs to change the flavor.

1. Set a large bowl next to the stove. In a large pot, mix together the wine, water, and lemon juice; bring to a boil. Poach the shrimp and sea scallops for 5 minutes. Remove to the bowl. Place the bluefish, turbot, scrod, or halibut into the water and allow to simmer for 4 minutes. Add to the bowl of seafood. Drop the crab leg pieces into the boiling water. Remove after 1 minute. Place in the bowl.

2. Poach the mussels until they open. Place in the bowl.

3. To the bowl, add the Italian dressing and the rest of the ingredients. Toss gently to coat. Refrigerate covered for 2 hours. Serve chilled or at room temperature.

>
> *Reduce the intake of calories here by making this salad a side dish for 4, or by reducing the amount of seafood in the recipe.*

Serves 4

PER SERVING

Calories: 553
GI: Low
Carbohydrates: 6 g.
Protein: 58 g.
Fat: 33 g.

¼ cup water
¼ cup dry white wine
1 teaspoon lemon juice
16 medium shrimp, raw, peeled, and deveined
16 medium sea scallops
½ pound filet of bluefish, turbot, scrod, or halibut, skinless
1 pound Alaskan crab legs, cut in 2-inch lengths, cracked
½ pound mussels, scrubbed
1 cup Italian dressing (see page 92)
2 teaspoons capers
Black pepper to taste
1 cup fresh Italian flat-leaf parsley, pulled from stems
½ teaspoon coriander seeds, cracked
1 teaspoon lemon zest
12 tiny currant tomatoes
½ red onion, thinly sliced

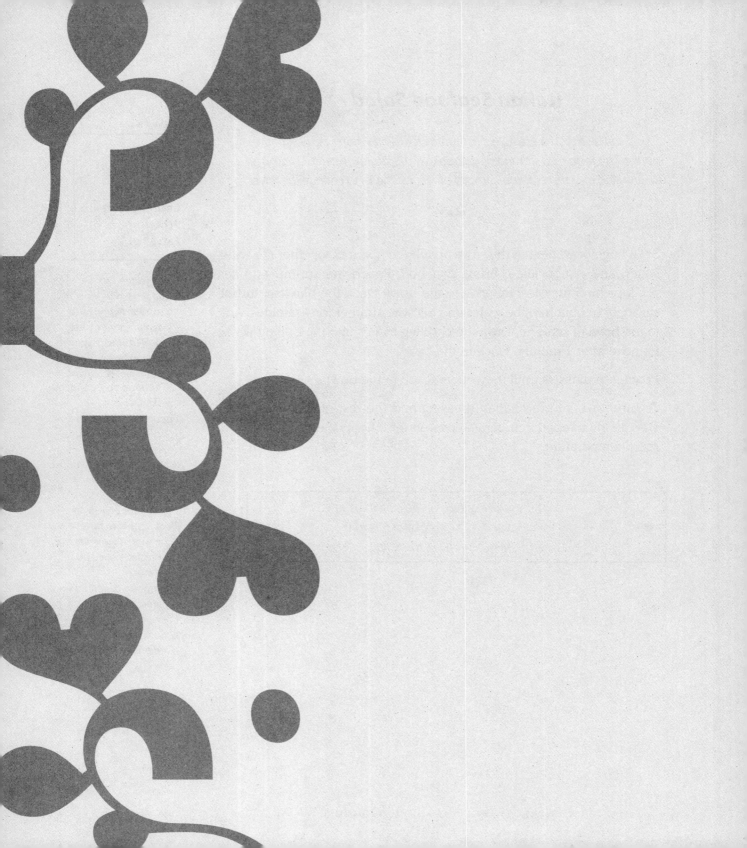

chapter 5
Soups

Asparagus Soup with a Float of Shrimp

This is a smooth and creamy soup with a slight bite from the Tabasco that is refreshing on a hot night. You could also serve it hot on a cold night.

Serves 2

PER SERVING

Calories: 332
GI: Very Low
Carbohydrates: 12 g.
Protein: 16 g.
Fat: 19 g.

½ pound asparagus, ends
    trimmed off, chopped
½ cup dry white wine
1-½ cups chicken broth
½ lemon, seeds removed
1 medium white onion,
    chopped
Tabasco sauce to taste
Salt and freshly ground black
    pepper to taste
½ cup whipping cream
6 medium shrimp, cooked,
    peeled, and deveined,
    chilled in the refrigerator

1. In a wide skillet, bring the white wine and chicken broth to a boil with the lemon and onion. Add asparagus and cook until tender. Add seasonings and whipping cream and remove lemon.

2. Purée everything but the shrimp in the blender.

3. Chill the soup until ready to serve. Pour into icy cold bowls. Float the shrimp on top of the soup and serve.

> In this soup, substitute whole or 2% milk
> for whipping cream.

Vegan Adaptations

If a soup recipe is for vegans, omit butter and use olive oil, use vegetable broth, and substitute soy milk for cream or regular milk.

Avocado Soup, Chilled with Lime Float

Most cold soups can also be served hot—avocado soup is an exception. Avocados can be delicious cooked, but this cold soup is too perfect to change.

1. In the blender, purée the avocados with chicken broth, buttermilk, lime juice, shallots, and salt. Taste for seasoning.

2. Whisk the sour cream, lime juice, lime zest, and Tabasco together. Float on top of the soup.

3. Serve icy cold.

> Substitute low-fat sour cream for regular sour cream. ❤

Zesty!

While zests are a fabulous way to add a kick of citrus flavor to almost any dish, be careful of lime zest—it gets very bitter when cooked. It is still a wonderful addition to fresh and uncooked dishes.

Serves 2

PER SERVING

Calories: 487
GI: Very Low
Carbohydrates: 23 g.
Protein: 6 g.
Fat: 45 g.

---

2 ripe avocados, peeled
½ cup chicken broth
½ cup buttermilk (nonfat is fine)
Juice of ½ lime
2 shallots, minced
½ teaspoon salt, or to taste
½ cup sour cream
1 teaspoon lime juice
Zest of ½ lime
Tabasco sauce to taste

Cold Basil and Fresh Tomato Soup

This is a wonderful summer soup, served cold, or heated for a cold day.
It is also good for you! The red tomatoes are full of vitamin C.
(The amount of vitamin C in tomatoes increases as they ripen.)
This soup also freezes beautifully!

Serves 4

PER SERVING

Calories: 60
GI: Very Low
Carbohydrates: 11 g.
Protein: 2 g.
Fat: 0 g.

2 pounds red, ripe tomatoes, halved and cored
1 cup beef broth
¼ cup red wine
1 teaspoon garlic powder
20 basil leaves
Salt and pepper to taste
Chopped chives for garnish

1. In the blender, purée tomatoes, beef broth, wine, garlic powder, basil, salt, and pepper. Chill overnight. Add garnish at the last minute.

2. If serving the soup hot, garnish with grated Cheddar or Parmesan cheese.

Cucumber Soup

Some recipes for cucumber soup call for cooking the cucumber.
This one "cooks" it in the acidity of lemon.

Serves 2

PER SERVING

Calories: 145
GI: Very low
Carbohydrates: 21 g.
Protein: 11 g.
Fat: 3 g.

1 slender, English cucumber, peeled and chopped
Juice of 1 lemon
1 cup nonfat buttermilk
1 cup low-fat yogurt
2 tablespoons fresh dill weed, snipped
Salt and freshly ground white pepper to taste
1 teaspoon Tabasco, optional
Garnish of extra snippets of dill or chives

1. Mix all ingredients together and purée in the blender until smooth. Place in a glass or other nonreactive bowl (to avoid staining a reactive bowl with the acidic citrus).

2. Let rest in the refrigerator for 4 hours or overnight.

3. Taste and add seasonings if necessary before serving in chilled bowls.

Black Bean Soup with Chilies

You can soak your black beans overnight and then cook for 2 to 3 hours or until tender. Canned beans also work well in this recipe. It's important to adjust the type of chilies to your personal taste. Serrano and Scotch bonnets are among the hottest.

1. In a large pot, fry the bacon. Remove bacon and leave the bacon fat in the pot. Add garlic, onion, and chilies to the pot. Sauté until softened, about 5 minutes.

2. Stir in the black beans, beef broth, tomato juice, rum, salt, and pepper. Cover and simmer for 1 hour.

3. You may either purée the soup or serve it as is. Garnish with any or all of the suggestions.

> *You have a few options to make this recipe more heart healthy. Instead of bacon, flavor the soup with a ham bone (which you must remove before puréeing or serving) or use vegetarian bacon.*

Serves 4

PER SERVING

Calories: 206
GI: Low
Carbohydrates: 27 g.
Protein: 11 g.
Fat: 5 g.

4 strips bacon, fried crisp, drained and crumbled
4 cloves garlic, chopped
1 medium sweet onion, chopped
2 hot chilies, seeded and minced
2 cans black beans or 1 pound black beans
8 ounces beef broth
½ cup tomato juice
2 ounces dark rum
Salt and black pepper to taste
Garnish of fresh lime wedges, sour cream, chopped cilantro, and pepper jack cheese

Broccoli Soup with Cheese

There is a lot to love about broccoli soup. Both nourishing and full of fiber, it can be enriched with cream or heated up with spicy pepper jack cheese.

Serves 4

PER SERVING

Calories: 297
GI: Very Low
Carbohydrates: 22 g.
Protein: 8 g.
Fat: 19 g.

¼ cup olive oil
1 medium sweet onion, chopped
2 cloves garlic, chopped
1 large baking potato, peeled and chopped
1 large bunch broccoli, coarsely chopped
½ cup dry white wine
3 cups chicken broth
Salt and pepper to taste
Pinch ground nutmeg
4 heaping tablespoons extra sharp Cheddar, grated, for garnish

1. Heat the olive oil in a large soup kettle. Sauté the onion, garlic, and potato over medium heat until softened slightly. Add the broccoli, liquids, and seasonings.

2. Cover the soup and simmer over low heat for 45 minutes.

3. Cool slightly. Purée in the blender. Reheat and place in bowls.

4. Spoon the cheese over the hot soup.

Save the Stalks

When you prepare broccoli, save the stems. They can be grated and mixed with carrots in a slaw, cut into coins and served hot, or cooked and puréed as a side. Broccoli marries well with potatoes and carrots and is good served raw with a dipping sauce.

Carrot Soup with Ginger

*The color of this soup looks especially seasonal in the fall or winter.
Be sure to get a fresh gingerroot for this recipe.
Its spicy flavor is warming on a chilly day.*

1. In a large pot, heat the olive oil and sauté the onion, celery, apple, and ginger. Add the carrots, chicken broth, salt, and a good grind of pepper.

2. Simmer the soup until the carrots are tender and the stock is reduced by 1 cup.

3. Purée in the blender and reheat. If adding cream, add to soup at this point.

Fabulous Celery

Celery is one of the most versatile vegetables. It goes in almost anything! It's great for dipping as well as stuffing. When you use celery as a dip with salsa, instead of chips, you go far lower on the GI scale. It's high in fiber and had almost no calories.

Serves 4

PER SERVING

Calories: 291
GI: Low
Carbohydrates: 13 g.
Protein: 3 g.
Fat: 29 g.

½ cup olive oil
1 large white onion, chopped
2 stalks celery, chopped
1 inch fresh gingerroot, peeled and chopped
4 large carrots, peeled and chopped
1 tart apple, peeled, cored, and chopped
4 cups chicken broth
Salt and freshly ground black pepper to taste
Options: ½ cup heavy cream, added when reheating the puréed soup

Carrot, Cauliflower, and Caraway Soup

For those of us who love the flavor of caraway seeds, this is wonderful!
If you don't care for that taste, simply omit the seeds.
For vegetarians, substitute vegetable broth or water for chicken broth.

Serves 4

PER SERVING

Calories: 194
GI: Low
Carbohydrates: 8 g.
Protein: 3 g.
Fat: 15 g.

1 teaspoon butter
¼ cup olive oil
½ sweet onion, chopped
½ head cauliflower
4 carrots, peeled and
     chopped
½ cup white vermouth or dry
     white wine
3-½ cups chicken broth
1 teaspoon caraway seeds
Salt and freshly ground black
     or white pepper to taste
1 teaspoon Worcestershire
     sauce
½ cup heavy cream

1. Using a large soup kettle, melt the butter and add olive oil over medium-low flame. Remove the core from the cauliflower and break into florets. Sauté the onion, cauliflower, and carrots for 4 to 5 minutes.

2. Add the white vermouth or wine, chicken broth, caraway seeds, salt, pepper, and Worcestershire sauce. Cover and simmer until the carrots and cauliflower are very tender.

3. Purée in the blender and reheat, adding the heavy cream just a few minutes before serving.

 Substitute heart-healthy margarine or olive oil for butter and replace heavy cream with whole or 2% milk.

Stretching Your Soup

It's best not to water soups down, unless you concentrate your soup before serving. To increase volume, you can add broth, canned tomatoes, wine, or extra veggies. You can also throw in leftover veggies and/or meat. You can also double or triple the recipes and freeze half or more.

Leek and Potato Soup (Hot or Cold)

There are many versions of this excellent soup, which tastes wonderful when served either hot or chilled. Some recipes have chunky potatoes, and others are smooth—you can prepare this one whichever way you prefer.

1. Heat the olive oil in a large soup kettle. Be sure to rinse the sand out of your leeks! Add the leeks and onion and sauté for 5 minutes over medium heat.

2. Add the potatoes, chicken broth, and salt. Simmer until the potatoes are tender. Set aside and cool.

3. Put the soup through a ricer or purée in the blender until smooth.

4. Pour the soup back into the pot, add the milk, whipping cream, and chives and reheat. Add salt and pepper to taste. Float the watercress on top for garnish.

 Replace 2% milk with nonfat milk.

Serves 4

PER SERVING

Calories: 491
GI: Moderate
Carbohydrates: 40 g.
Protein: 8 g.
Fat: 33 g.

¼ cup olive oil
2 leeks, coarsely chopped
1 large sweet onion, chopped
2 large baking potatoes, peeled and chopped
2 cups chicken broth
1 teaspoon salt
1 cup 2% milk
1 cup whipping cream
¼ cup chopped chives
Salt and freshly ground pepper to taste
Garnish of ¼ cup chopped watercress

Onion Soup with Poached Egg Float

This makes a wonderful midnight supper.
Make the soup in advance, and then after heating it, add the eggs.

Per Serving

Calories: 392
GI: Very Low
Carbohydrates: 23 g.
Protein: 9 g.
Fat: 15 g.

2 tablespoons olive oil
½ sweet red onion, chopped
½ sweet white onion,
    chopped
2 shallots, chopped
2-¾ cups rich beef broth
2 tablespoons port wine
1 teaspoon Worcestershire
    sauce
1 bay leaf
Salt and pepper to taste
4 eggs

1. Heat the olive oil in a large saucepan. Add the onions and shallots. Sauté for 6 minutes. Add the beef broth, wine, bay leaf, and Worcestershire sauce. Cover and reduce heat to low. Simmer for 30 minutes.

2. Add salt and pepper to taste. You can chill the soup until just before serving.

3. Heat the soup. Carefully drop in the eggs and poach for 2 minutes. Serve soup with eggs floating on top.

Onions, Shallots, and Chives

When it comes to onions, the more varieties the merrier! When you use several different varieties, you get a depth of flavor that would not be possible if you just use one kind of onion—so mix it up!

Egg Drop Soup with Lemon

This is a lovely spicy version of the Chinese staple, made with a variety of Asian sauces. Asian fish sauce is a liquid made from salted fish that is used in place of salt in many Asian recipes. Hoisin sauce is made from crushed soybeans and garlic, has a sweet and spicy flavor, and is a rich brown color.

1. Heat the peanut oil in a large saucepan. Sauté the garlic over medium heat until softened, about 5 minutes.

2. Add chicken broth, lemon juice, hoisin sauce, soy sauce, fish sauce, chili oil, and gingerroot. Stir and cover. Cook over low heat for 20 minutes.

3. Just before serving, whisk the eggs with a fork. Add to the boiling soup and continue to whisk until the eggs form thin strands.

Serves 2

PER SERVING

Calories: 158
GI: Very Low
Carbohydrates: 2 g.
Protein: 5 g.
Fat: 13 g.

1 tablespoon peanut oil
1 clove garlic, minced
2 cups chicken broth
Juice of ½ lemon
1 tablespoon hoisin sauce
1 teaspoon soy sauce
1 teaspoon Asian fish sauce
½ teaspoon chili oil, or to taste
1 inch fresh gingerroot, peeled and minced
2 eggs

Old-Fashioned New England Oyster Stew

*This is one of the most comforting of comfort foods,
especially if you come from New England. Be careful not to overcook
the oysters! A good guideline is to cook them until the edges curl.*

Per Serving

Calories: 222
GI: Very Low
Carbohydrates: 17 g.
Protein: 13 g.
Fat: 12 g.

1 tablespoon butter
1 shallot, minced
1 stalk celery, minced
1 tablespoon quick-blending
    flour (such as Wondra)
1 cup 2% milk
1 cup clam broth (bottled or
    dried is fine)
1 teaspoon Worcestershire
    sauce
Pinch ground nutmeg
½ pint shucked oysters,
    drained, juice reserved
Pepper to taste

1. Melt the butter in a large saucepan. Over medium-low heat sauté the shallot and celery until soft. Stir in the flour, milk, and clam broth. Add the Worcestershire sauce and nutmeg.

2. When the soup is steaming but not boiling, gently ladle in the oysters and grind some pepper into the soup. Skip the salt—there is salt in the clam broth and oysters. When very hot, but not boiling, serve.

> *Substitute nonfat milk for 2% milk. Use olive oil or
> heart-healthy margarine for butter.*

Yellow Pepper and Tomato Soup

*Yellow peppers and yellow tomatoes are very sweet
and make a wonderful soup!*

1. In a soup kettle, heat the oil over medium flame and sauté the onion, garlic, and yellow pepper. After about 5 minutes add the chicken broth and tomatoes.

2. Stir in the seasonings, lemon juice, salt, and pepper.

3. Cover and simmer. You can purée the soup if you wish or leave some bits of texture in it.

4. Serve hot or cold and sprinkle with basil.

Colorful Veggies

Yellow fruits and vegetables are loaded with vitamin A, or retinol, which keeps your skin moist and helps your eyes adjust to changes in light.

Serves 4

PER SERVING

Calories: 176
GI: Very Low
Carbohydrates: 12 g.
Protein: 2 g.
Fat: 14 g.

¼ cup peanut oil
1 sweet yellow bell pepper, seeded, finely chopped
½ cup sweet white onion, chopped
2 cloves garlic, minced
1-½ cups chicken broth
4 medium-sized yellow tomatoes, cored and puréed
½ teaspoon cumin, ground
½ teaspoon coriander, ground
Juice of ½ lemon
Salt and pepper to taste
Garnish of fresh basil leaves, torn

Spinach and Sausage Soup with Pink Beans

*This is a hearty and delicious soup. If you don't want
to work with fresh spinach, get a package of frozen, chopped spinach.
You can also substitute escarole or kale. Some sausage is so lean
that you will need to add a bit of oil when you cook it.*

Serves 4

PER SERVING

Calories: 344
GI: Very Low
Carbohydrates: 28 g.
Protein: 19 g.
Fat: 20 g.

8 ounces Italian sweet
    sausage, cut in bite-size
    chunks
¼ cup olive oil
2 white onions, chopped
4 cloves garlic, chopped
2 stalks celery, chopped,
    leaves included
2 cups beef broth
2 cups water
Bunch fresh spinach, kale,
    or escarole, or 10-ounce
    package frozen, chopped
    spinach
1 teaspoon dried oregano
1 teaspoon red pepper flakes
13-ounce can pink or red
    kidney beans, drained
Salt to taste
Grated Parmesan cheese

1. Place the sausage in a soup kettle. Add ¾ cup water and bring to a boil; let water boil off. Add the oil if dry and sauté the onions, garlic, and celery for 10 minutes over medium-low heat.

2. Stir in the rest of the ingredients except the cheese; cover and simmer for 35 minutes. Serve in heated bowls. Garnish with grated Parmesan cheese.

❤ *Substitute vegetarian sausage for regular sausage.* ❤

Lentil Soup with Winter Vegetables

This is a substantial soup that will get you through a long winter!

Put all ingredients in a soup kettle, bring to a boil, cover, and simmer for 1 hour.

Serves 4

PER SERVING

Calories: 188
GI: Low
Carbohydrates: 19 g.
Protein: 18 g.
Fat: 5 g

½ pound bag red or yellow lentils
4 cups vegetable broth
2 cups water
2 parsnips, peeled and chopped
2 carrots, peeled and chopped
2 white onions, chopped
4 cloves garlic, chopped
4 small bluenose turnips, peeled and chopped
½ pound deli baked ham, cut in cubes

Pumpkin Soup (Slightly Sweet)

If you have a sweet tooth, you can add some more brown sugar to this recipe.

Stir the ingredients into the soup pot, one-by-one, whisking after each addition. Cover and simmer for 10 minutes. If you decide to use the cream, add at the last minute.

Serves 4

PER SERVING

Calories: 102 *(with heavy cream, add 100 calories)*
GI: Low
Carbohydrates: 24 g.
Protein: 4 g.
Fat: 0 g.

1 cup Vidalia or other sweet onion, finely chopped
½ inch fresh gingerroot, peeled and minced
2 cups orange juice
2 cups chicken broth
13-ounce can pumpkin (unflavored)
1 teaspoon brown sugar
½ teaspoon ground cinnamon
¼ teaspoon ground nutmeg
¼ teaspoon ground cloves
Optional: ½ cup heavy cream

Mediterranean Seafood Soup

This is a quick and easy soup that will give you a taste of the Mediterranean.

Serves 2

PER SERVING

Calories: 450
GI: Very Low
Carbohydrates: 19 g.
Protein: 48 g.
Fat: 18 g.

2 tablespoons olive oil
½ cup sweet onion, chopped
2 cloves garlic, chopped
½ bulb fennel, chopped
2 cups tomatoes, chopped
½ cup dry white wine
1 cup clam broth (canned is fine)
6 littleneck clams, tightly closed
6 mussels, tightly closed
8 raw shrimp, jumbo, peeled and deveined
1 teaspoon dried basil, or 5 leaves fresh basil, torn
Salt and red pepper flakes to taste

1. Heat the oil over medium flame and add onion, garlic, and fennel. After 10 minutes, stir in the wine and clam broth and add the tomatoes. Bring to a boil.

2. Drop clams into the boiling liquid. When clams start to open, add the mussels. When mussels start to open put in the shrimp, basil, salt, and pepper flakes. Serve when shrimp turns pink.

Littleneck Clams

Littleneck clams are the smallest variety of hard-shell clams and can be found on the northern east and west coasts of the United States. They have a sweet taste and are delicious steamed and dipped in melted butter, battered and fried, or baked.

Pumpkin Soup (Savory)

*Pumpkin soup is fine any time of year. You can always use
canned pumpkin, which is very good and easier than peeling
and cooking fresh pumpkin. Be sure to buy unsweetened and unflavored
pumpkin so that you don't end up with soup tasting like pumpkin pie!*

1. Melt the butter in a soup kettle and sauté the onion over medium-low heat for 5 minutes. Stir in all but the heavy cream and ham.

2. Simmer the soup, covered for 10 minutes. Add heavy cream and serve hot with ham sprinkled on top.

> Substitute olive oil for butter and
> whole milk for heavy cream.

Serves 4

Per Serving

Calories: 166
GI: Low
Carbohydrates: 9 g.
Protein: 2 g.
Fat: 13 g.

1 teaspoon butter
1 cup yellow onion, chopped
1-½ cups chicken broth
¼ cup dry white wine
1 teaspoon sage leaves, dried,
    or 4 fresh sage leaves,
    chopped
½ teaspoon oregano, dried
2 cups canned pumpkin
    (unflavored)
Salt to taste
1 teaspoon Tabasco sauce
Garnish of chopped fresh
    chives
½ cup heavy cream
Garnish with ⅛ pound
    smoked ham, chopped

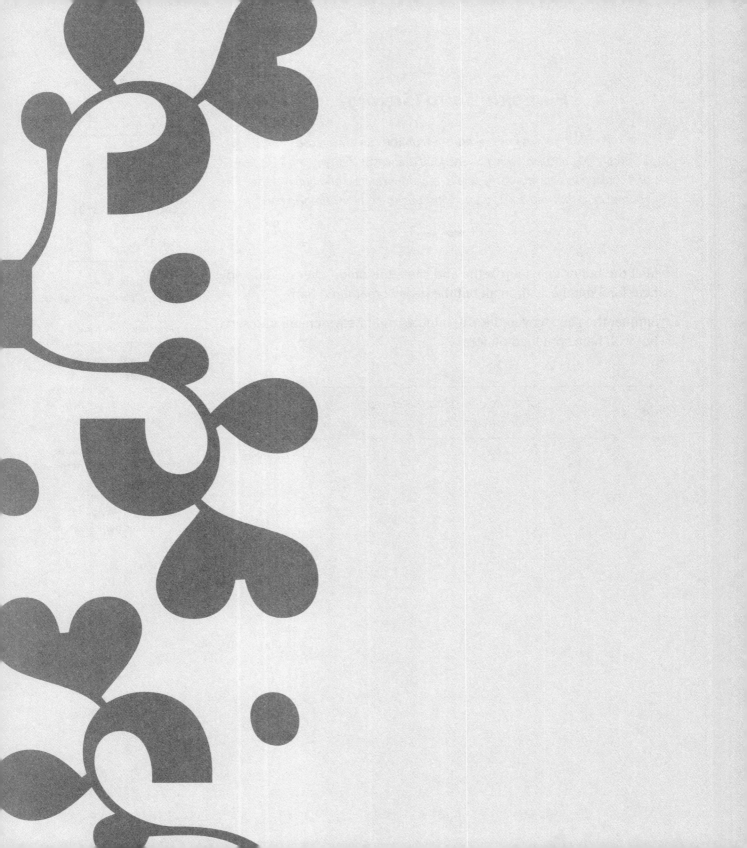

chapter 6
Healthy Snacks and Dips

Broiled Herb-Crusted Chicken Tenders

Chicken tenders are always popular with kids, and you can try this for entertaining adults, too. The skewers make the chicken tenders easy and fun for kids to eat with their hands and make these chicken tenders a convenient appetizer for a party.

1. Preheat broiler to 400°F. Rinse the chicken tenders and pat dry. Mix the olive oil, herbs, salt, and pepper. Dip the chicken tenders in this mixture.

2. Skewer each piece of herbed chicken tender and broil on a baking sheet for 3 minutes per side. Serve with any of the dipping sauces in this chapter.

Apple-Cheddar Melts on Pita Toast

A nice crisp apple is essential for this snack so that it won't turn mushy in the oven. Granny Smiths work well in this recipe, as do Empire and Ginger Gold apples.

1. Preheat the broiler to 400°F. Toast one side of the pita. Cut in quarters.

2. Stack the apple slices and cheese slices on each pita piece. Place back under the broiler until cheese melts.

Whole Wheat Pita Bread

Whole wheat pita bread stands up well to toasting and has a nutty and delicious flavor. You can also stuff it with any number of goodies and then bake it. Try pita toast instead of crackers as bases for various snacks.

Pita Toast with Herbs and Cheese

These pita toast snacks are an easy alternative to traditional appetizers. They work equally well as after school snacks for kids and starters for a cocktail party.

Toast the pitas and cut in fourths. Using a fork, mix the rest of the ingredients together in a small bowl. Spread on pitas and serve.

Makes 4 snacks

PER SERVING

Calories: 77
GI: Low
Carbohydrates: 9 g.
Protein: 4 g.
Fat: 5 g.

1 whole wheat pita
2 tablespoons cream cheese, at room temperature
2 teaspoons Gorgonzola cheese, at room temperature
2 sprigs fresh parsley, minced
2 tablespoons chives, minced
Salt and pepper to taste

Bagel Chips

You can buy bagel chips in the supermarket, but they are usually so hard you could break your teeth. Try these instead!

1. Thinly slice the bagels crosswise, discarding the tiny ends.

2. Spread the pieces on a baking sheet. Spray with olive oil and sprinkle with garlic salt and pepper.

3. Bake at 350°F for 10 minutes. Serve as crackers.

Makes 12 chips

PER SERVING

Calories: 26
GI: Low
Carbohydrates: 5 g.
Protein: 1 g.
Fat: 0 g.

2 whole wheat or pumpernickel bagels
Spray bottle of olive oil
Garlic salt and pepper to taste

Creamy-Crunchy Avocado Dip with Red Onions and Macadamia Nuts

This is one of the best dips you can make. Try it with bagel chips, pita toast, or even good corn chips.

Using a small bowl, mash the avocado and mix in the rest of the ingredients. Serve chilled.

Serves 2

PER SERVING

Calories: 229
GI: Zero
Carbohydrates: 10 g.
Protein: 3 g.
Fat: 22 g.

1 large ripe avocado, peeled, pit removed
Juice of ½ fresh lime
2 tablespoons red onion, minced
2 tablespoons macadamia nuts, chopped
1 teaspoon Tabasco or other hot red pepper sauce
Salt to taste

Rice Cakes

Serve hot or cold and with a sweet or pungent sauce.

1. Cool the cooked rice. Beat the egg, sugar, cinnamon, and salt together. Mix into the rice.

2. In a frying pan, heat the oil to 350°F and fry cakes until golden. Serve hot or cold.

Makes 4 cakes

PER SERVING

Calories: 194
GI: Moderate
Carbohydrates: 12 g.
Protein: 2 g.
Fat: 15 g.

1 cup cooked rice, basmati or arborio
1 egg
1 teaspoon sugar
Cinnamon to taste (start with ¼ teaspoon)
¼ teaspoon salt, or to taste
¼ cup canola oil

Parmesan Tuilles

These are too tasty and easy to be true! They make excellent cocktail snacks to go with dry martinis or ginger ale.

Grate the cheese, using a box grate on its coarsest side. Heat the oil in a well-seasoned frying pan or a nonstick pan and drop small mounds of the cheese onto the pan, flattening with the back of a spoon. Fry for 2 minutes per side. Serve hot or cold, garnished with paprika.

Makes 6 tuilles

PER SERVING

Calories: 36
GI: Very Low
Carbohydrates: 0 g.
Protein: 2 g.
Fat: 4 g.

6 tablespoons fresh Parmesan cheese
2 teaspoons canola oil
Sprinkle of paprika

Black Bean Dip

This is excellent for parties or as a snack and is also very low in fat.

Pulse all ingredients in the food processor or blender. Serve chilled or at room temperature.

> ❤ *Substitute low-fat sour cream for regular sour cream.* ❤

Makes 2 cups

PER SERVING

Calories: 283
(18 calories per 1-ounce serving)
GI: Low
Carbohydrates: 39 g.
Protein: 12 g.
Fat: 13 g.

1-½ cups black beans, canned and drained
½ cup Vidalia onion, finely minced
4 cloves garlic, minced
2 teaspoons red hot pepper sauce, or to taste
Juice of 1 lime
½ cup sour cream
½ cup chopped cilantro or parsley
Salt and pepper to taste

Grilled Stuffed Cherry Tomatoes

*These grilled tomatoes can be prepared and served hot or
kept uncooked and refrigerated for the next day.*

Serves 4
(4 tomatoes per person)

PER SERVING

Calories: 177
GI: Very Low
Carbohydrates: 28 g.
Protein: 5 g.
Fat: 6 g.

---

16 large cherry tomatoes
3 tablespoons mascarpone
  cheese, at room
  temperature
1 teaspoon oregano
Salt and pepper to taste
Olive oil in a spray bottle

1. Rinse the tomatoes. Cut off the top ¼ of the ball and save to use as hats. Leave stems on. Using the small end of a melon baller, remove the seeds and pulp from the insides of the tomatoes.

2. Mix the mascarpone, oregano, salt, and pepper with a fork. Push the cheese mixture into the tomatoes. Pop the "hats" on top.

3. Spray the tomatoes with olive oil.

4. Place on a hot grill for 2 to 3 minutes, moving to heat all sides or do not grill but simply refrigerate and serve cold.

Homemade Hummus

*Garlic lovers can add more garlic to this popular Middle Eastern dip. You can
buy hummus at the store, but this recipe is easy to make and much cheaper.*

Makes 1-½ cups, serves 12

PER SERVING

Calories: 128
GI: Low
Carbohydrates: 9 g.
Protein: 2 g.
Fat: 9 g.

15-ounce can chickpeas,
  drained
2 cloves garlic, chopped, or
  to taste,
½ small white onion,
  chopped
1 teaspoon Tabasco or other
  hot sauce
½ cup fresh flat-leaf parsley,
  or cilantro, tightly packed
Salt and black pepper to taste
½ cup olive oil

Blend all ingredients in the food processor or blender. Do not purée—you want a coarse consistency. Serve with bagel chips or warm pita bread.

All Natural Olive Oil Spray

To make your own olive oil spray, you can buy a clean spray bottle at a hardware store and fill it with olive oil. If using a spray bottle from your house, make sure it has never contained anything that could leave a harmful residue. Use this spray as an alternative to nonstick sprays that don't taste like olive oil.

Polenta Cubes with Salsa

Polenta cubes are crunchy and good for snacks or as croutons on salads.

1. Stir the cornmeal in a fine stream into boiling salted water. Cook, stirring for about 20 minutes or until the polenta comes away from the sides of the pan. Add Parmesan cheese and chives. Prepare a 9" × 9" glass baking pan with nonstick spray and spread the polenta in the pan.

2. Chill the polenta. When polenta is firm, turn it out onto waxed paper and cut into 1-inch cubes.

3. Fry the cubes at high heat, turning as the sides brown. Drain on paper towels and serve with salsa.

Makes 80 1-inch cubes

PER SERVING (PER CUBE)

Calories: 19
GI: Moderate
Carbohydrates: 1 g.
Protein: 1 g.
Fat: 1 g.

3 cups water
1 cup yellow corn meal
1 teaspoon salt
½ cup Parmesan cheese
½ cup chives, finely minced
½ cup canola oil
Salsa (see below)
Nonstick spray

Salsa

*Like many Spanish and Mexican-influenced dishes
that Americans love, this salsa is versatile and easy to make.
If you want super heat in the salsa, include the pepper seeds.
You can also substitute hot chili sauce or hot red pepper flakes.*

1. Drop the tomatoes in boiling water for 3 minutes. Drain, cool, slip off skins, and chop into a medium-sized bowl.

2. Mix in the rest of the ingredients. Let rest for 2 hours in the refrigerator; serve.

Makes 1 cup

PER SERVING

Calories: 153
(19 calories per 1-ounce serving)
GI: Very Low
Carbohydrates: 36 g.
Protein: 5 g.
Fat: 0 g.

4 medium-sized tomatoes
½ cup red onion, chopped
2 cloves garlic, minced
*1 serrano chili, seeded and
    minced, or more to taste*
Juice of ½ lime
½ cup cilantro, chopped
Salt and pepper to taste

Green Salsa

*This Mexican classic is delicious in omelets or used as a dip
and provides an alternative to the usual red salsa you find in America.
Add more jalapeños for some extra heat.*

Place all ingredients in the blender and pulse until coarsely chopped.
Rest in refrigerator for 2 hours. Serve chilled.

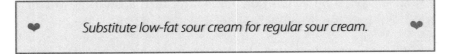

Substitute low-fat sour cream for regular sour cream.

Tomatillo Tutorial

*Tomatillos are husked tomatoes that look like green tomatoes when
their papery husk is removed. You can find them in most major supermarkets. Choose unblemished tomatillos that fully fill out their husks.*

Makes 1 cup

PER SERVING

Calories: 332
(40 calories per 1-ounce serving)
GI: Very Low
Carbohydrates: 24 g.
Protein: 0 g.
Fat: 24 g.

---

6 tomatillos, chopped, husks
   discarded
4 cloves garlic, minced
2 jalapeño peppers, cored
   and chopped, seeds
   included
½ cup sour cream
½ cup cilantro
Salt to taste

Sour Cream and Gorgonzola Dip for Crudités

Perhaps the healthiest of snacks is a plate of raw veggies and a low-cal dip like this one.

Pulse all ingredients in the food processor or blender; serve chilled with a selection of raw vegetables.

Makes 1-½ cups

PER SERVING

Calories: 268
(22 calories per 1-ounce serving)
GI: Zero
Carbohydrates: 6 g.
Protein: 8 g.
Fat: 24 g.

¾ cup low-fat sour cream
¼ cup Gorgonzola cheese,
    crumbled
½ teaspoon celery salt
1 teaspoon Tabasco or other
    hot sauce
2 tablespoons lemon juice

Creamy Spiced Dip for Crudités

This recipe is a tasty way to get the right amounts of vitamin-loaded veggies into your diet.

Pulse all ingredients in the food processor or blender. Serve cold with a selection of raw vegetables.

Makes 1 cup

PER SERVING

Calories: 496
(62 calories per 1-ounce serving)
GI: Zero
Carbohydrates: 14 g.
Protein: 0 g.
Fat: 48 g.

½ cup low-fat mayonnaise
½ cup low-fat sour cream
¼ cup fresh parsley, chopped
4 scallions, chopped
1 teaspoon curry powder
1 tablespoon fresh lime juice
Salt and hot red pepper flakes
    to taste

Mango Salsa

This is excellent with shrimp, crab legs, or fruit.
Avoid using frozen mango since it tends to be mushy when thawed.

Pulse all ingredients in the food processor or blender. Turn into a bowl, chill, and serve.

Makes 1 cup

PER SERVING

Calories: 209
(26 calories per 1-ounce serving)
GI: Low
Carbohydrates: 54 g.
Protein: 2 g.
Fat: 0 g.

1 mango, peeled and diced
¼ cup sweet onion, minced
2 teaspoons cider vinegar
2 jalapeño peppers, cored,
    seeded, and minced
Juice of ½ lime
2 tablespoons cilantro or
    parsley, finely chopped
Salt to taste

Dip for Fresh Fruit

This is excellent with slices of apple, pineapple, or pear.
Enjoy with any seasonal fruit.

Blend all ingredients in the blender. Serve chilled.

Makes 1-½ cups

PER SERVING

Calories: 239
(20 calories per 1-ounce serving)
GI: Zero
Carbohydrates: 8 g.
Protein: 11 g.
Fat: 15 g.

4 ounces low-fat cream cheese
4 ounces low-fat cottage
    cheese
1 teaspoon sugar substitute,
    or to taste
1 teaspoon freshly ground
    white pepper
2 tablespoons cider vinegar
    or lemon juice
½ teaspoon salt, or to taste

Pineapple Chutney

Serve on the side with chicken, pork, or seafood.

In a medium-sized bowl, mix all ingredients together. Cover and refrigerate, letting the flavors develop for 2 hours.

Makes 2 cups

PER SERVING

Calories: 60
(4 calories per 1-ounce serving)
GI: Very Low
Carbohydrates: 15 g.
Protein: 0 g.
Fat: 0 g.

1-½ cups fresh pineapple, diced
2 tablespoons fresh mint,
    chopped
1 tablespoon curry powder
Juice of ½ lime
1 teaspoon cider vinegar
Salt to taste

Peanut and Fruit Sauce

This is wonderful for dipping grilled shrimp, chicken, or pork.

Pulse all ingredients in the food processor or blender. Let rest for 2 hours, covered in the refrigerator. Return to room temperature just before serving.

Makes 1 cup, serves 20

PER SERVING

Calories: 67
GI: Low
Carbohydrates: 2 g.
Protein: 3 g.
Fat: 6 g.

¾ cup peanut butter
1 tablespoon soy sauce
1 teaspoon sesame oil
Juice of 1 lime
4 scallions, chopped
1 tablespoon fresh cilantro,
    chopped
1 tablespoon hot chili sauce
1 tablespoon Worcestershire
    sauce
Salt to taste

**Makes 1 cup
(2 tablespoons per serving)**

PER SERVING

Calories: 63
GI: Zero
Carbohydrates: 0 g.
Protein: 0 g.
Fat: 7 g.

⅓ cup balsamic vinegar
½ teaspoon dry mustard
1 teaspoon lemon juice
2 cloves garlic, chopped
1 teaspoon oregano, dried,
    or 1 tablespoon fresh
    oregano leaves
Salt and pepper to taste
½ cup extra-virgin olive oil

**Makes 1 cup
(2 tablespoons per serving)**

PER SERVING

Calories: 77
GI: Zero
Carbohydrates: 1 g.
Protein: 0 g.
Fat: 9 g.

⅓ cup red wine vinegar
½ teaspoon Worcestershire
    sauce
1 clove garlic, chopped
2 tablespoons fresh parsley,
    chopped
1 teaspoon thyme, dried
1 teaspoon rosemary, dried
Pinch sugar
⅔ cup extra-virgin olive oil

Italian Dressing

*Try doubling this recipe and storing in a glass jar.
It will keep for several days and is much better than supermarket dressings.*

Put all but the olive oil into the blender and blend until smooth. Whisk in the oil slowly in a thin stream. Bottle and give it a good shake before you use it!

French Dressing

*This is a great dressing on a crisp green salad.
You can also use it as a marinade for beef, chicken, or pork.*

Mix all ingredients except the olive oil in the blender. Slowly add the oil in a thin stream so that the ingredients will emulsify.

Balsamic Vinaigrette and Marinade

*Because balsamic vinegar is very sweet, it needs a slightly
sour counterpoint. In this case, it is lemon juice. It also needs a bit of zip
like pepper or mustard. Use this recipe as a dressing or a marinade.*

Place all but the olive oil in the jar of the blender. With the blender running on a medium setting, slowly pour the oil into the jar. Blend until very smooth. Cover and store in the refrigerator for up to 7 days.

The Condiment of Kings

Mustard is one of the oldest condiments, having been used for over 3,000 years! The first mustards were made from crushed black or brown mustard seeds mixed with vinegar. In 1856, the creator of Dijon mustard, Jean Naigeon, changed the recipe into what it is today—crushed mustard seeds mixed with sour juice made from unripe grapes.

**Makes 1 cup
(2 tablespoons per serving)**

PER SERVING

Calories: 76
GI: Zero
Carbohydrates: 4 g.
Protein: 0 g.
Fat: 7 g.

---

*2 cloves garlic, minced
2 shallots, minced
⅓ cup balsamic vinegar
Juice of ½ lemon
Salt and pepper to taste
½ teaspoon Dijon-style
  mustard
½ cup olive oil*

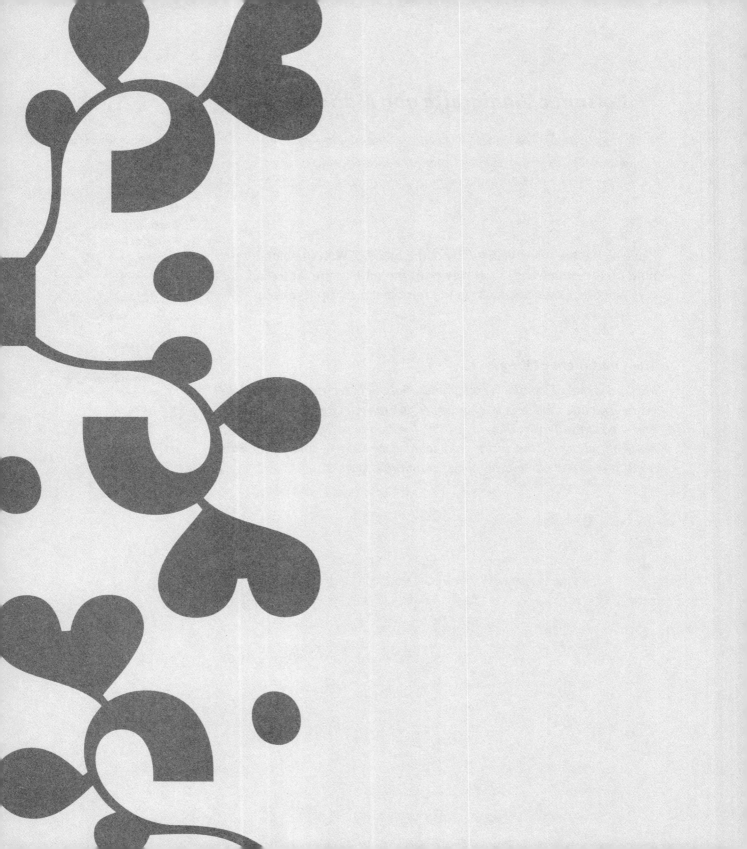

chapter 7
Sandwiches

Sausage and Peppers with Melted Mozzarella Cheese

This classic Italian combination is usually served as a sub or hero.
Try it on thinly sliced whole wheat bread and use less sausage and peppers.

Makes 2 sandwiches

PER SERVING

Calories: 295
GI: Low
Carbohydrates: 36 g.
Protein: 25 g.
Fat: 8 g.

¼ pound Italian sausage link,
   cut in 8 pieces
½ cup sweet white onions,
   thinly sliced
4 thin slices whole wheat or
   sourdough bread
4 slices red roasted peppers
   (from a jar is fine)
4 thin slices mozzarella
   cheese
2 teaspoons Italian dressing
   (see page 92)
½ cup shredded Napa
   cabbage or romaine
   lettuce

1. Fry sausage slices in a nonstick pan over low heat. When brown, drain on paper towels.

2. Add the onions and sizzle over low heat until wilted; reserve.

3. Toast the bread. Place the sausage slices on two pieces of toast. Arrange the onions, peppers, and cheese.

4. Run under a hot broiler until the cheese melts. Pile with shredded cabbage or lettuce for crunch.

> Substitute vegetarian sausage for regular sausage
> and use low-fat cheese.

Baby Eggplant with Tomato

Baby eggplants are great to cook with because they don't take very long to grill or sauté and are never bitter. You can get dark purple, mauve, or white ones, all of which are wonderful. Baby eggplants are tender enough so that you can leave the skins on when you grill or sauté them.

1. Preheat the broiler to 400°F. Place the cut pieces of eggplant in a bowl. Coat with Italian dressing. Place on a baking sheet, sprinkle with Parmesan cheese, and run under the broiler until golden on both sides.

2. Sprinkle tomato slices with basil, oregano, salt, and pepper.

3. Stack the eggplant and tomato on toast, top with another piece of toast, and enjoy!

Sweat Your Eggplant

Eggplant is a member of the nightshade family and is related to tomatoes and potatoes. If eggplant is a little overripe (which happens often with larger eggplant), it will have a bitter taste. To get rid of bitter taste, place sliced eggplant in a colander and sprinkle with salt. Allow the eggplant to "sweat" for 20 minutes and rinse before using.

Serves 2

PER SERVING

Calories: 200
GI: Low
Carbohydrates: 33 g.
Protein: 10 g.
Fat: 7 g.

2 baby eggplants, the size of jumbo eggs, stem ends trimmed, cut crosswise in ¼ inch slices
2 tablespoons Italian dressing (see page 92)
2 teaspoons Parmesan cheese
1 tomato, sliced
1 teaspoon basil, dried
1 teaspoon oregano, dried
4 slices whole wheat bread, toasted
Salt and pepper to taste

Turkey Parmesan

Leftover turkey is great for whipping up quick lunches. This sandwich's melted Parmesan sets it apart from the usual post-Thanksgiving turkey sandwich.

Makes 2 sandwiches

PER SERVING

Calories: 251
GI: Low
Carbohydrates: 29 g.
Protein: 22 g.
Fat: 8 g.

2 slices turkey breast
4 slices whole wheat bread
4 teaspoons low-fat mayonnaise
2 teaspoons Parmesan cheese
1 teaspoon thyme leaves, dried
Salt and pepper to taste
Shredded lettuce or Napa cabbage

1. Set your broiler on 400°F. Toast 4 slices of bread.

2. Mix the mayonnaise, cheese, thyme, salt, and pepper. Spread the mixture on one side of the bread.

3. Run under the broiler. Plate the toast and place turkey on two slices. Finally, add shredded lettuce or Napa cabbage for crunch and close sandwiches.

For the Kids— Peanut Butter and Banana with Jam

This recipe is great for kids. They love the sweetness of bananas and jam, and the whole wheat crackers are nutritious!

2 servings

PER SERVING

Calories: 167
GI: Moderate
Carbohydrates: 25 g.
Protein: 5 g.
Fat: 7 g.

8 whole wheat crackers
4 teaspoons peanut butter
1 banana, cut in 8 slices
1 teaspoon raspberry jam or jelly

Place ½ teaspoon of peanut butter on each cracker. Top with banana slices and a dab of jelly on each.

Hot and Spicy Pork Meatball Sub

*Pork makes excellent meatballs. Spiked with pepper and barbeque sauce,
you have wonderful sandwiches.*

1. Mix the pork, salt, pepper, cloves, Tabasco sauce, chili sauce, and egg in a bowl.

2. Form 16 small meatballs and roll them in the bread crumbs. Heat the oil to 350°F and fry meatballs until brown and crisp all over.

3. Drain the meatballs on paper towels. Place on rolls, drizzle with barbeque sauce, and pile with onions.

> *To cut back on calories in this recipe, you can make this serve six people instead of four. Make 18 smaller meatballs instead of 16 larger ones and serve them on 6 rolls.*

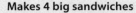

Makes 4 big sandwiches

PER SERVING

Calories: 541
GI: Low
Carbohydrates: 29 g.
Protein: 29 g.
Fat: 34 g.

1 pound ground pork
Salt and pepper to taste
¼ teaspoon ground cloves
1 tablespoon Tabasco sauce
2 tablespoons chili sauce
1 egg, well beaten
½ cup fine bread crumbs
½ inch canola oil in a heavy
frying pan
4 teaspoons of your favorite
barbeque sauce
½ sweet onion, thinly sliced
4 hero rolls (whole wheat if
possible)

Broiled Swordfish Club

Makes 2 sandwiches

PER SERVING

Calories: 419
GI: Low
Carbohydrates: 29 g.
Protein: 39 g.
Fat: 18 g.

4 slices lean bacon or turkey
 bacon
2 swordfish filets, about
 5 ounces each
2 tablespoons lemon juice
Salt and pepper to taste
2 teaspoons low-fat
 mayonnaise
1 teaspoon dried dill, or
 2 teaspoons fresh dill
 weed
4 slices whole grain bread
8 thin slices cucumber
4 slices fresh tomato

*Who says you need three slices of bread to make a club sandwich?
What you do need is two slices of whole grain bread per sandwich.*

1. Fry the bacon and drain on a paper towel. Sprinkle the fish with lemon juice, salt, and pepper. Run under a hot (450°F) broiler for 3 minutes per side.

2. Mix the mayonnaise and dill. Spread on the bread. Stack the bacon, fish, cucumber, and tomato on two slices of bread. Finish with top slice and cut. Serve with crunchy cucumber slices.

> Substitute Canadian bacon or
> vegetarian bacon for regular bacon.

Fresh Fish and Seafood Sandwiches

Because items like swordfish, tuna, shrimp, and other seafood cook so quickly, they are ideal for a fast sandwich. During the summer, cook your shrimp the night before and refrigerate it, or you can buy precooked and shelled shrimp, trading flavor for convenience.

Grilled Vegetable and Three Cheese Panini

A panini is a grilled sandwich with a heavy weight on top to squish it down. You can use a heavy frying pan or foil-covered brick on top!

1. Brush eggplant and squash with Italian dressing and grill. Grill red pepper, skin side to flame until it chars. Place red pepper, while still hot, in a plastic bag. The skin will come right off! Sprinkle veggies with Parmesan cheese and set aside.

2. Spread both sides of 4 pieces of bread with Italian dressing. Load with vegetables and Muenster and Gorgonzola cheeses.

3. Place panini on lightly oiled fry pan or panini press. If using a fry pan, cover it with a second pan or foil-covered brick. Toast the sandwich on medium heat until very brown. Turn if using a frying pan.

4. Cut sandwiches and serve piping hot!

Makes 2 Sandwiches

PER SERVING

Calories: 459
GI: Low
Carbohydrates: 48 g.
Protein: 23 g.
Fat: 24 g.

¼ cup Italian dressing (see page 92)
2 baby eggplants, thinly sliced
½ yellow summer squash, cut in ¼ inch coins
1 sweet red pepper, cored and seeded
2 teaspoons Parmesan cheese, grated
4 slices Tuscan bread (try to get whole wheat or sourdough)
2 slices Muenster cheese, thinly sliced
2 teaspoons Gorgonzola cheese, crumbled
Oil for panini press or frying pan

Smoked Salmon and Mascarpone Stuffed Pita Pockets

This recipe is a wonderful mixture of textures, melted and soft on the inside and slightly crisp on the outside.

Serves 2

PER SERVING

Calories: 302
GI: Very Low
Carbohydrates: 36 g.
Protein: 13 g.
Fat: 13 g.

2 whole wheat pita pockets
2 thin slices of red onion
2 thin slices of lemon, seeded
⅛ pound smoked salmon
⅛ pound mascarpone
　cheese, sliced
1 teaspoon green peppercorns,
　packed in brine
Black pepper to taste

1. Preheat the oven to 350°F. Using half of each ingredient, stuff the pockets with onion, lemon, salmon, cheese, and peppercorns.

2. Bake for 15 to 20 minutes, until the pita is golden and the filling is hot.

Fresh Tuna and Wasabi Mayonnaise Grinder

*Wasabi is Japanese horseradish and very, very spicy.
It is delicious when used wisely!*

Makes 2 sandwiches

PER SERVING

Calories: 571
GI: Low
Carbohydrates: 41 g.
Protein: 35 g.
Fat: 30 g.

8-ounce fresh tuna steak
Salt and pepper
¼ cup mayonnaise
½ teaspoon wasabi powder,
　or to taste
10 green beans
4 slices tomato, thinly sliced
Sourdough whole wheat
　French bread, cut in 5-
　inch lengths and split

1. Salt and pepper the tuna steak. Sear on a nonstick pan over medium flame. Blanch green beans for 3 minutes in boiling water; chop. Mix the mayonnaise and wasabi powder; add the chopped beans.

2. When the tuna is medium rare, about 4 minutes per side, slice it thinly. Stack with the mayonnaise-bean mixture and tomatoes on the bread. Serve immediately.

> ❤ *Replace regular mayonnaise with low-fat mayonnaise.* ❤

Shrimp and Cucumber Tea Sandwich

These are perfect as a lunch or cut into small bites for cocktail snacks.

1. Place the shrimp, cream cheese, onion, and dill in the food processor or blender. Pulse until well mixed, but not puréed.

2. Spread the shrimp mixture on the bread. Sprinkle with salt and pepper and top with cucumber slices. Finish with final slice of bread and cut in diamonds.

Tea Time

Tea sandwiches are small and dainty in order to stave off hunger until dinner time. Traditionally, tea sandwiches are served on thinly sliced, buttered white bread lightly spread with a cream cheese or mayonnaise-based mixture and topped with fresh vegetables.

Makes 2 sandwiches

PER SERVING

Calories: 164
GI: Low
Carbohydrates: 16 g.
Protein: 17 g.
Fat: 5 g.

4 slices extra thin whole wheat bread, crusts trimmed
¼ pound shrimp, cooked
2 tablespoons low-fat cream cheese, at room temperature
2 tablespoons sweet onion, chopped
½ teaspoon dill, dried, or 1 tablespoon fresh dill
Salt and pepper to taste
8 slices cucumber

Sautéed Crab Cake and Avocado Wraps

Lots of cooks use surimi (imitation crabmeat) for crab cakes because crab meat can be expensive. Substituting large cabbage leaves for bread in this recipe keeps the GI down.

Makes 4 thick wraps

PER SERVING

Calories: 245
GI: Low
Carbohydrates: 7 g.
Protein: 18 g.
Fat: 17 g.

10-ounce package imitation
    crabmeat
4 tablespoons low-fat
    mayonnaise
1 teaspoon Dijon-style
    mustard
1 egg
Salt and pepper to taste
⅛ inch canola oil in frying
    pan
4 large cabbage leaves
1 avocado, peeled and sliced
    around pit
4 slices fresh lemon, paper-
    thin
Garnish with extra lemon
    wedges and parsley
    sprigs

1. Lightly mix the crabmeat, mayonnaise, mustard, egg, salt, and pepper. Set a heavy pan over medium heat and coat the bottom with canola oil. Form cakes and sauté until well browned on both sides.

2. Blanch cabbage leaves in boiling water and then shock in cold water to stop cooking.

3. Lay out the cabbage leaves. Use a fork to mash the avocado and dab on the cakes. Roll cabbage leaves to make wraps. Decorate with lemon and place a crab cake on each. Garnish with extra lemon wedges and parsley sprigs.

Thanksgiving Wraps

You don't have to wait for Turkey Day leftovers to enjoy these!

1. Toss all but the lettuce together in a large bowl.

2. Lay out the lettuce leaves, add turkey filling, and roll them up.

Cranberry Additions

Dried cranberries make a tasty addition to many everyday foods. Add them to cereal, trail mix, oatmeal cookies, chocolate chip cookies, and salads for a sweet and tart surprise.

Makes 12 small wraps

PER SERVING

Calories: 89
GI: Low
Carbohydrates: 3 g.
Protein: 11 g.
Fat: 3 g.

2 cups cooked turkey, diced
1 stalk celery, minced
½ cup red seedless grapes, halved
2 tablespoons red onion, minced
¼ cup dried cranberries
6 tablespoons low-fat mayonnaise
1 teaspoon dried thyme
Salt and pepper to taste
12 large romaine lettuce leaves

Easter Monday Wraps

This is an excellent way to use up the extra ham from Easter dinner.

Serves 2

PER SERVING

Calories: 567
GI: Low
Carbohydrates: 34 g.
Protein: 32 g.
Fat: 30 g.

4 large corn tortillas
¼ cup low-fat mayonnaise
½ teaspoon curry powder
1 teaspoon mustard
2 teaspoons cider vinegar
2 green onions, chopped
⅔ cup baked ham, chopped
1 green apple, peeled, cored, and chopped
½ cup Monterey Jack cheese, cubed

1. Preheat oven to 350°F. Whisk together mayonnaise, curry powder, mustard, cider vinegar, and green onions in a bowl.

2. Add the ham, apple, and cheese, folding to coat.

3. Lightly toast tortillas. Mound the mixture on the tortillas, wrap, and serve as is or bake for 10 minutes.

Monterey Jack

Some sources attribute the name of Monterey Jack cheese to a Scottish immigrant turned wealthy landowner and dairy farm owner named David Jacks, who settled in Monterey, California in the mid-1800s. Others say that the name originated from the use of presses or "jacks" in the cheese production process.

Melted Gorgonzola and Asparagus in Corn Tortillas

*While the creamy melted Gorgonzola cheese in this recipe
makes it taste luxurious, these wraps are still full of nice green veggies!
Remember that the darker green the vegetable, the more vitamins
and minerals it contains.*

1. Heat the olive oil over medium setting. Add onion and asparagus and cook, stirring for 10 minutes. Remove from the heat and add the cheese and pepper.

2. Using a grill or griddle that you've prepared with nonstick spray, toast the tortillas on one side. Turn and spread with the asparagus and cheese mixture. Fold in half and brown lightly on both sides.

Serves 2

PER SERVING

Calories: 154
GI: Very Low
Carbohydrates: 18 g.
Protein: 9 g.
Fat: 7 g.

1 teaspoon olive oil
1 tablespoon sweet onion,
*   minced*
½ of one 10-ounce box
*   frozen asparagus spears,*
*   thawed and chopped*
1 ounce Gorgonzola cheese
Black pepper to taste
2 corn tortillas
Nonstick spray

Grilled Pork and Mango Salsa Sandwich

*Perhaps the nicest cut of pork is the tenderloin. It cooks quickly and pairs well
with fruits such as mangos, pineapples, apples, and peaches.*

1. Using the corn muffin mix, follow the directions for corn bread. Bake; cut into 8 squares (2" × 2").

2. Sprinkle the pork tenderloin with soy sauce, salt, and pepper.

3. Heat a heavy frying pan and add the peanut oil. Sauté the pork for 8 minutes per side or until medium, turning frequently. When done, let the pork rest for 8 to10 minutes. Slice thinly on a diagonal.

4. Place 2 pieces of corn bread on serving plates. Stack slices of pork on each. Top with mango salsa.

Serves 4

PER SERVING

Calories: 371
GI: Low to Moderate
*(depending on the thickness of
the corn bread)*
Carbohydrates: 16 g.
Protein: 39 g.
Fat: 17 g.

1 package corn muffin mix
1 pound pork tenderloin,
*   trimmed*
2 tablespoons soy sauce
Salt and pepper to taste
2 tablespoons peanut oil
½ cup mango salsa (see page
*   90)*

Buffalo Mozzarella with Greek Olives and Roasted Red Peppers

Mixing textures enhances flavors—the creaminess of the mozzarella is a nice counterpoint to the salty tang of the olives.

Makes 12 small sandwiches

Per Serving

Calories: 58
GI: Low
Carbohydrates: 11 g.
Protein: 4 g.
Fat: 1 g.

4 ounces buffalo mozzarella, thinly sliced
½ cup Greek olives, pitted and chopped
½ cup jarred red roasted peppers packed in olive oil, chopped
2 tablespoons red wine vinegar
3 large whole wheat pitas

1. Mix the chopped olives and red peppers with the vinegar. Push the mozzarella and vegetables into the pita pockets.

2. Place on a baking sheet. Bake at 350°F until golden brown, about 15 minutes.

3. When browned and hot, cut sandwiches in quarters and serve.

Buffalo Mozzarella

Unlike most available mozzarella cheese, which is made from cow's milk, buffalo mozzarella is made from the milk of water buffalo. Since buffalo milk contains far more butterfat than cow's milk, the result is a much creamier cheese that is still slightly elastic and mild like other fresh mozzarella cheese.

chapter 8
Pasta, Polenta, and Sauces

Asparagus and Cheese Sauce for Rotini

*Asparagus in a cheese sauce with bits of ham and scallions
is a terrific seasonal spring dish.*

Serves 4

PER SERVING

Calories: 633
(including pasta)
GI: Low
Carbohydrates: 90 g.
Protein: 33 g.
Fat: 16 g.

1 pound rotini pasta
½ pound asparagus, cut in
    1-inch lengths
2 tablespoons olive oil
½ large white onion, chopped
2 cloves garlic, chopped
¼ pound smoked ham or
    prosciutto, chopped
1 teaspoon thyme, dried
1 cup ricotta (nonfat milk
    is fine)
1 egg, beaten
½ cup parsley, chopped
4 tablespoons Parmesan
    cheese, grated
Nonstick spray

1. Cook pasta, drain it, and place in a baking dish that you have prepared with nonstick spray.

2. Preheat oven to 350°F. Heat the olive oil and sauté the garlic and onion until softened. Blanch asparagus for 5 minutes in boiling water; add along with thyme and ham to sautéed garlic and onion. Mix and remove from heat.

3. Mix the ricotta, egg, and parsley and combine with asparagus mixture. Gently fold into the rotini in baking dish and sprinkle with Parmesan cheese.

4. Bake for 20 minutes and serve.

Shocking!

To keep green vegetables green after cooking, shock them in ice-cold water after boiling or blanching. Then, give them a quick toss in butter or oil for beautifully green vegetables. This works well with beans, broccoli, asparagus, and other greens.

Caper, Egg, and Prosciutto Sauce for Orecchiette

Orecchiette are tiny, ear-shaped pasta.
(The Italian word for ear is orecchio.) You could always use
spaghetti with this or any other pasta you have on hand.

Serves 4

PER SERVING

Calories: 663
(including pasta)
GI: Low
Carbohydrates: 84 g.
Protein: 26 g.
Fat: 24 g.

1 pound orecchiette
¼ cup olive oil
2 cloves garlic, chopped
¼ cup parsley
1 teaspoon dried oregano, or
   2 teaspoons fresh
3 tablespoons capers
⅛ pound prosciutto,
   shredded
4 eggs, well beaten
Salt and pepper to taste
4 tablespoons Parmesan
   cheese, grated

1. While the pasta is cooking, heat the olive oil in a heavy frying pan. Sauté the garlic over medium heat for 5 minutes. Stir in the parsley, oregano, and capers. Remove from the heat.

2. When the pasta is done, drain it and place in a large, warm, serving bowl. Toss in the herbs, capers, prosciutto, and garlic mixture. Then, stir in the beaten eggs, tossing to cook.

3. Sprinkle with Parmesan cheese, and salt and pepper to taste.

Prosciutto

Prosciutto is a dry cured ham made by salting a leg of pork and leaving it to cure for about two months. After the salting period, the pork is hung in a sunny, breezy place for a time, after which it is moved to an airy room and is left to age, often for a year or more.

Grilled Vegetable Sauce for Spaghetti

*Grilled vegetables, brushed with olive oil and herbs,
make an excellent sauce for your favorite pasta.*

Serves 4

PER SERVING

Calories: 580
(including pasta)
GI: Low
Carbohydrates: 96 g.
Protein: 20 g.
Fat: 13 g.

*2 baby eggplants, stemmed
and sliced in ⅓ inch coins*
*1 medium zucchini, stem
removed and cut
lengthwise in ⅓ inch
pieces*
*1 yellow pepper, cored,
seeded, cut in quarters*
4 medium tomatoes, halved
*¼ cup balsamic vinaigrette
(see page 93)*
*2 tablespoons extra-virgin
olive oil*
4 cloves garlic, chopped
8 fresh basil leaves, torn
Salt and pepper to taste
*1 pound of your favorite
pasta*
Garnish of Parmesan cheese

1. Set the grill on high. Brush the vegetables with the balsamic vinaigrette. Grill until just done, about 3 minutes per side. Grill tomatoes on a piece of aluminum foil.

2. Cook the pasta. In a large frying pan, heat the olive oil and sauté the garlic over medium heat. Coarsely chop the vegetables and add to the sautéed garlic. Chop the tomatoes and add.

3. Stir in the basil, salt, and pepper. Drain the pasta into a serving bowl and stir in the vegetables. Garnish with extra pepper and plenty of Parmesan cheese.

Handling Cooked Pasta

Many chefs undercook pasta slightly and add it to the sauce in the pan. This way, the pasta absorbs flavors from the sauce. Remember that if you put pasta into a hot pan of sauce, it will continue to cook—be careful not to overcook and end up with mush!

Pasta with Tomato and Black Olive Sauce

*If you can get grape or currant tomatoes, they are wonderful;
otherwise, use cherry tomatoes and cut them in half. Anchovies can
add a subtle and delicate flavor to a sauce or salad dressing.
Try buying them in paste that comes in a tube.*

1. While the pasta is cooking, heat the olive oil in a large frying pan. Add the garlic and scallions and cook over low heat until wilted. Mash the anchovies into the oil. Add the tomatoes and wine.

2. Raise heat and bring to a boil. Reduce heat and simmer for 10 to 12 minutes.

3. Stir in the rest of the ingredients. Drain the pasta. Place pasta in a bowl, stir in the sauce, and serve hot!

Serves 2

PER SERVING

Calories: 695 *(including pasta)*
GI: Low
Carbohydrates: 87 g.
Protein: 29 g.
Fat: 23 g.

½ pound of your favorite
    pasta
2 tablespoons olive oil
2 cloves garlic, minced
4 scallions, chopped
3 anchovies
1 teaspoon red pepper flakes,
    or to taste
½ pint grape or cherry
    tomatoes, cut in halves
½ cup dry white wine
1 teaspoon dried oregano
½ cup Italian or Greek
    black olives, pitted and
    chopped
½ cup fresh Italian flat-leaf
    parsley, chopped
½ cup Parmesan cheese,
    grated

Spring Green Peas and Ricotta Sauce for Baked Ziti

Mixing ricotta and peas is classic in Italian cuisine.
Baby bells are smaller versions of portobello mushrooms.
If you don't want to shell fresh peas,
buy a box of frozen baby peas and enjoy.

Serves 4

PER SERVING

Calories: 752 *(including pasta)*
GI: Low
Carbohydrates: 92 g.
Protein: 59 g.
Fat: 15 g.

1 pound ziti
¼ cup olive oil
10 baby bell mushrooms
    or Italian brown
    mushrooms, sliced
6 scallions, chopped
½ cup frozen baby peas
1-½ cups ricotta cheese
1 egg, beaten
Pinch nutmeg
Salt and pepper to taste
½ cup smoked ham, finely
    chopped
1 pound raw shrimp, peeled
    and deveined
¼ cup Parmesan cheese,
    grated
Nonstick spray

1. While the pasta is cooking, sauté the mushrooms and scallions in olive oil for 10 minutes over medium heat. Add the peas and stir, letting them defrost.

2. Preheat oven to 350°F. Remove the pan from the heat and stir in the ricotta, egg, nutmeg, salt, and pepper. Stir in the ham. Drain the pasta and place in a baking dish that you have prepared with nonstick spray. Stir in the cheese mixture.

3. Mix the shrimp into the casserole and sprinkle with Parmesan cheese. Bake for 20 minutes.

White Clam Sauce for Linguini

*If you have had this with canned clams and liked it,
you'll love it with fresh clams!*

1. Salt the water and set it on to boil for the linguini. Scrub the clams under cold, running water. Make sure all are tightly closed and discard any cracked clams. Tap two clams together. If you hear a hollow or dull sound, one is dead. You should hear a sharp click.

2. Heat olive oil and sauté the garlic over medium flame. When the garlic is soft, pour in the clam broth and white wine. Bring to a boil. Put the clams into the boiling liquid.

3. Drain the pasta and place in a bowl. When the clams open, they are ready. Serve clams whole with plenty of red pepper flakes, oregano, and parsley.

Wine Pairing

You may want to serve Pinot Grigio with this dish. Called Pinot Gris in France, it is a medium-bodied, somewhat sweet and acidic white wine that especially complements seafood.

Serves 2

PER SERVING

Calories: 654 *(including pasta)*
GI: Low
Carbohydrates: 87 g.
Protein: 31 g.
Fat: 18 g.

½ pound linguini
18 littleneck clams
2 tablespoons extra-virgin olive oil
2 cloves garlic, chopped
1 cup clam broth (bottled or powdered is fine)
¼ cup dry white wine
½ teaspoon oregano, dried
1 teaspoon red pepper flakes, or to taste
½ cup Italian flat-leaf parsley, chopped

Peppery Red Mussel Sauce for Linguini

Mussels produce the most delicious broth, so they are great in sauce and soups. Today, most mussels that you buy commercially are farm-raised and don't have shaggy beards and lots of sand. Also called Mussels Fra Diavolo, this dish is wonderful for a family dinner or an elegant supper.

Serves 4

PER SERVING

Calories: 581 *(including pasta)*
GI: Low
Carbohydrates: 94 g.
Protein: 28 g.
Fat: 8 g.

1 pound whole wheat linguini
3 pounds fresh mussels
1 tablespoon unsalted butter
2 cloves garlic, minced
¼ cup sweet onion, chopped
1 teaspoon lemon rind, finely ground
Juice of ½ lemon
½ cup dry white wine
2 cups plum tomatoes (crushed or canned is fine)
Salt, if needed
1 tablespoon red pepper flakes

1. Set a large pot of salted water on the stove for the pasta. After scrubbing the mussels, tap them together and listen for a sharp click. Discard any that sound hollow.

2. Heat the butter in a large soup pot. Sauté the garlic and onion over medium heat. Add the lemon rind and lemon juice after five minutes.

3. Stir in the wine and tomatoes, salt, if needed, and pepper flakes. Bring to a boil. Cover and simmer for 10 minutes.

4. Drain the pasta and place in a large serving bowl. Put the mussels into the sauce pot. Return to a boil; as soon as the mussels start to open, use tongs to put them over the pasta. Throw away any mussels that do not open. Pour the sauce over the mussels and pasta.

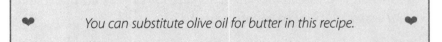

You can substitute olive oil for butter in this recipe.

Shrimp and Spinach Sauce for Pasta

*This dish makes it easy to get both your vitamins
and your protein in one dish. Shrimp cooks quickly,
in about 2 minutes, depending on the kind of heat you are using.
In a sauté pan, cook for 1 minute per side,
on a hot grill, 30 seconds per side.*

1. While the pasta is cooking, heat the olive oil in a large saucepan. Sauté the garlic over medium heat. Add the lemon juice, spinach, shrimp, and seasonings. Stir until the spinach wilts and the shrimp turns pink.

2. Drain the pasta and turn into a serving bowl. Mix in the sauce and sprinkle with Parmesan cheese. Serve immediately.

Preparing Fresh Shrimp

Why go to all the trouble of peeling and deveining shrimp? The reasons are flavor and texture. The vein you remove is largely harmless but usually contains grit or sand that would ruin your meal. Ready-to-eat shrimp are already deveined, but they have less flavor than fresh shrimp.

Serves 4

PER SERVING

Calories: 619 *(including pasta)*
GI: Low
Carbohydrates: 88 g.
Protein: 41 g.
Fat: 11 g.

1 pound of your favorite pasta
2 tablespoons olive oil
4 cloves garlic, chopped
Juice of ½ lemon
1 bag baby spinach, chopped
1 pound raw shrimp, peeled and deveined
Pinch nutmeg
½ teaspoon cayenne pepper
Salt to taste
4 teaspoons Parmesan cheese, grated

Anchovy, Garlic, and Olive Sauce for Pasta

This is truly Italian comfort food!

Serves 2

PER SERVING

Calories: 552 *(including pasta)*
GI: Low
Carbohydrates: 84 g.
Protein: 16 g.
Fat: 17 g.

½ pound angel hair pasta
2 teaspoons unsalted butter
1 tablespoon olive oil
2 cloves garlic, chopped
1 inch anchovy paste
10 black olives, pitted
½ cup fresh parsley, chopped
Freshly ground black pepper

1. Make the sauce while the pasta is cooking. Melt the butter over medium heat, add olive oil, and sauté the garlic for 3 minutes.

2. Whisk the anchovy paste, parsley, and pepper into the butter and garlic. Toss sauce with olives and pasta.

3. If too dry, add some of the pasta water.

Pesto for Angel Hair Pasta

The combination of basil, garlic, pine nuts, and olive oil is classic and delicious. In the old days, Italians used a mortar and pestle to make this uncooked basil sauce. For our purposes, a blender works just as well. Make the sauce in advance and cook the angel hair pasta at the last minute.

Serves 4, as a side

PER SERVING

Calories: 466 *(including pasta)*
GI: Very Low
Carbohydrates: 5 g.
Protein: 8 g.
Fat: 50 g.

4 cloves garlic
½ cup olive oil
½ cup pine nuts (pignoles)
    (can substitute walnuts)
2 cups basil leaves, stemmed
    and packed into
    measuring cup
Salt and pepper to taste
½ cup Parmesan cheese,
    grated
Angel hair pasta

1. Spread the pine nuts on a baking sheet and lightly toast under the broiler.

2. Place the garlic and olive oil in blender and blend until chopped. Add the rest of the ingredients a bit at a time until you have the consistency of coarse cornmeal. Serve over hot angel hair pasta or polenta.

Basic Polenta with Butter and Cheese

In some parts of Italy, polenta is used more than pasta! It is simply cornmeal cooked in boiling water until soft and fluffy like mashed potatoes. When polenta is cooled, it stiffens up, making it useful for frying or grilling. This classic can be used instead of pasta or potatoes. Serve as a base for stews, veggies, or pasta sauces.

1. Bring the water to a boil. Add salt. Stir in the cornmeal in a thin stream, stirring constantly. Reduce heat to low; continue to stir for 20 minutes or until the polenta comes away from the pot.

2. Stir in the butter, cheese, pepper, and parsley.

Serves 4

PER SERVING

Calories: 68
GI: Moderate
Carbohydrates: 6 g.
Protein: 2 g.
Fat: 4 g.

3-½ cups water
1 teaspoon salt
1 cup yellow cornmeal, coarsely ground
1 tablespoon butter or heart-healthy margarine
2 tablespoons Parmesan or Fontina cheese, grated
Pepper to taste
Garnish with parsley

Polenta with Broccoli Rabe

Broccoli rabe is a leafy vegetable whose florets resemble those of broccoli. It packs a wonderful and slightly bitter, acidic punch that contrasts with the mildness of the polenta.

1. Rinse the broccoli rabe and cut in 1-½ inch pieces, trimming off very bottoms of stems.

2. Drop the broccoli rabe into the boiling water and cook for 5 minutes. Shock in cold water. Drain thoroughly.

3. Heat the olive oil and add garlic; sauté over medium heat for a few minutes; add the lemon juice, pepper flakes, and drained broccoli rabe. Cook and stir until well coated.

4. Serve over hot polenta.

Serves 4

PER SERVING

Calories: 74
GI: Low
Carbohydrates: 3 g.
Protein: 1 g.
Fat: 7 g.

Basic polenta recipe (see above)
1 pound broccoli rabe
1 quart boiling, salted water
2 tablespoons olive oil
2 cloves garlic, minced
Juice of ½ lemon
Red pepper flakes to taste

Sautéed Polenta Patties
with Italian Tuna

Try this for lunch on a hot day or supper on a warm night.

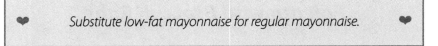

Serves 4

PER SERVING

Calories: 333
GI: Moderate
Carbohydrates: 7 g.
Protein: 14 g.
Fat: 29 g.

*Basic polenta recipe
    (see page 119)
1 pound green beans
Juice of 1 lemon
¼ cup mayonnaise
2 cans of tuna, drained
    (imported, Italian tuna if
    you can find it)
4 polenta patties
¼ cup olive oil
Salt and pepper to taste
Nonstick spray*

1. Chill polenta in an 8" × 10" glass pan that you have prepared with nonstick spray. Cool the polenta until very firm, at least 3 hours in the refrigerator.

2. Blanch the green beans and shock. Drain and reserve. Mix the mayonnaise and lemon juice in a small bowl.

3. Sauté 4 polenta patties in olive oil over medium heat. Place on individual serving plates. Add tuna and green beans. Add salt and pepper to taste.

4. Drizzle with the lemon and mayonnaise mixture and serve.

> ❤ *Substitute low-fat mayonnaise for regular mayonnaise.* ❤

White Bean, Tomato, and Zucchini Sauce for Polenta or Pasta

Since pasta is made of semolina flour, which is a low GI carbohydrate, it has a lower GI level than polenta. Try to find coarsely ground cornmeal for polenta because it breaks down more slowly.

1. Start the pasta or polenta. In a large pan over medium heat, sauté garlic, zucchini, and onions. When softened, add the rest of the ingredients. Cover, reduce heat, and simmer for 15 to 20 minutes.

2. Spoon sauce over polenta or pasta. Garnish with parsley.

Polenta Possibilities

Polenta is boiled, slow-cooked cornmeal that can be made into different consistencies depending on the purpose you would like it to serve in your meal. Using less water, you can make polenta like cornbread and grill it, or you can add more water to make thinner polenta that you can serve with sauce, meat, or cheese and treat like pasta.

Serves 4

PER SERVING (SAUCE ONLY)

Calories: 274
GI: Low
Carbohydrates: 27 g.
Protein: 8 g.
Fat: 14 g.

1 pound pasta or basic polenta recipe (see page 119)
¼ cup olive oil
3 cloves garlic, minced
½ cup sweet onions, chopped
1 tablespoon rosemary leaves, dried or 2 tablespoons fresh
2 cups tomatoes, crushed or chopped (canned are fine)
15-ounce can large white beans, drained
1 medium zucchini, trimmed and diced
1 teaspoon oregano, dried
6 fresh basil leaves, torn
¼ cup beef broth
Salt and pepper to taste
Garnish of fresh parsley, chopped

Sausage and Escarole Sauce for Polenta or Pasta

Serves 4

PER SERVING
(SAUCE ONLY)

Calories: 234
GI: Zero
Carbohydrates: 6 g.
Protein: 24 g.
Fat: 13 g.

Basic polenta recipe (see page 119) or 1 pound pasta
1 pound Italian sausage, sweet or hot, cut in bite-size pieces
2 cloves garlic, minced
Olive oil, if needed
¼ cup dry white wine
1 cup Italian plum tomatoes, crushed or chopped (canned are fine)
2 cups escarole, torn into small pieces
1 teaspoon oregano, dried
1 teaspoon thyme, dried
Salt and pepper to taste
½ cup fresh parsley
½ cup Parmesan or Fontina cheese, grated

If you skip the pasta or polenta, you can easily turn this into an excellent soup by adding chicken or beef broth.

1. Prepare the polenta or pasta. In a heavy deep frying pan, fry the sausage over medium heat. If very lean, add some water. Stir in the garlic when the sausage is almost done. If the pan is dry, moisten with a bit of olive oil.

2. Add the rest of the ingredients, with the exception of the cheese. Cover and reduce heat to a simmer. Simmer for 15 minutes or until the escarole wilts. Add cheese immediately before serving.

> *You can substitute vegetarian sausage for regular sausage in this recipe.*

The Endive's Cousin

Escarole is a relative of endive and has loose, wavy leaves. The outer leaves have a much more bitter taste, so use the milder inner leaves for salads. Be sure to wash carefully since escarole traps grit and dirt between its leaves while growing!

Vegetable Lasagna with Buffalo Mozzarella

This dish accomplishes the goal of making both vegetarians and meat-eaters pleased with what you serve. This vegetable lasagna will feed a crowd and satisfy any type of guest!

1. While cooking the lasagna noodles (undercook a bit to avoid soggy lasagna), heat the oil in a large sauce or frying pan over medium flame. Sauté the vegetables for 10 minutes, adding the herbs, salt, and pepper at the end.

2. Preheat oven to 325°F. In a large bowl, mix the ricotta, Parmesan cheese, and eggs. Mix in the vegetables. Prepare a 9" × 13" lasagna pan with nonstick spray.

3. Cover the bottom with sauce and then with strips of cooked lasagna. Spoon the ricotta and vegetable mixture over the pasta. Cover with a second layer of lasagna and repeat until you get to the top of the pan.

4. Spread the final layer of lasagna with sauce. Bake for 35 minutes. Five minutes before serving, dot the top with the mozzarella. When it melts, serve.

Serves 10

PER SERVING

Calories: 414
GI: Low
Carbohydrates: 44 g.
Protein: 22 g.
Fat: 18 g.

1 package lasagna
¼ cup olive oil
1 fresh zucchini, cut in thin coins
1 cup broccoli florets, cut in small pieces
1 yellow pepper, cored, seeded, and diced
½ pint grape tomatoes, cut in halves
6 scallions, chopped
10 fresh basil leaves, torn
¼ cup fresh parsley, chopped
Salt and pepper to taste
2 pints ricotta cheese
½ cup Parmesan cheese, grated
2 eggs, beaten
2 cups of your favorite pasta sauce
5 ounces buffalo mozzarella
Nonstick spray

Pumpkin-Filled Ravioli

*This is a savory way to make use of wonton wrappers.
Serve with butter or chicken gravy. You can also place the
uncooked ravioli on a baking sheet and freeze. When frozen,
place them in a plastic bag and store for an easy supper!*

Serves 4

PER SERVING

Calories: 130
GI: High
Carbohydrates: 36 g.
Protein: 11 g.
Fat: 5 g.

10 ounces canned pumpkin
1 egg
*¼ cup Parmesan cheese,
    grated*
Salt and pepper to taste
*1 teaspoon savory leaves,
    dried*
½ teaspoon sage
2 teaspoons butter, melted
24 wonton wrappers
Nonstick spray

1. Using the electric mixer, beat together the first 7 ingredients. Lay out the wonton wrappers. Spoon filling on one side of each.

2. Dipping your finger in cold water, moisten the edges of the wonton wrappers and press together, making sure edges are tightly sealed.

3. Prepare a 4-quart pot of boiling, salted water. Cook the ravioli until they rise to the surface; serve hot with butter, sauce, or gravy.

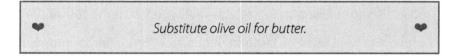

Substitute olive oil for butter.

Sicilian Seafood Sauce for Rice or Pasta

Sicily is surrounded by water and populated by seafood lovers. Fish, shellfish, and southern vegetables are dietary staples of this beautiful Italian island.

1. Heat the olive oil in a large pot. Add the vegetables and cook until softened, about 15 minutes. Stir in wine, sugar, herbs, and clam broth. Bring to a boil; reduce heat to a simmer. Cover and cook for 1 hour.

2. Return to a boil and add the lobster and clams. After 5 minutes, put the mussels on top. When the mussels begin to open, add the squid and shrimp. Serve as soon as the shrimp turns pink, about 2 to 3 minutes.

Cooking Seafood in Proper Sequence

It is important to start with the items that take the longest to cook. Lobster and clams take longer than mussels, which take about 6 to 8 minutes. Shrimp, scallops, and squid cook within 2 to 3 minutes. If you do put the shrimp, scallops, and squid in with the lobster, clams, or mussels, they will be chewy and tough.

Serves 4

PER SERVING

Calories: 338
GI: Zero
(pasta/rice not included)
Carbohydrates: 17 g.
Protein: 30 g.
Fat: 18 g.

¼ cup olive oil
½ fennel bulb, about ⅔ cup, trimmed and chopped, save tops for garnish
1 red onion, chopped
4 cloves garlic, chopped
¼ cup dry red wine, full-bodied, such as Chianti
Pinch sugar
2 sprigs fresh oregano, stripped from stems
10 fresh basil leaves
1 cup clam broth
28-ounce can chopped tomatoes
1 lobster in shell (claws, tail, and body), cut in chunks, head discarded
12 littleneck clams
12 mussels
2 squid, about 4 inches each, cut in rings
12 medium shrimp

Gramolata, Tuscan Garnish

This fabulous garnish is an all-purpose flavor maker! Sprinkle it on soups, pasta, polenta, or rice. It is fabulous over seafood stew.

Use a blender or mortar and pestle to combine ingredients. Blend all ingredients and spoon lightly over just about anything.

Makes ½ cup

**Per Serving
(10 servings)**

Calories: 71
GI: Zero
Carbohydrates: 0 g.
Protein: 0 g.
Fat: 8 g.

*Juice and rind of 1 lemon
2 cloves garlic, chopped
½ cup stemmed, loosely
    packed parsley
Salt and red pepper flakes to
    taste
3 ounces olive oil*

Short Ribs of Beef over Polenta

This is an easy, Italian way of making those nice fat, meaty spareribs.

1. Using a large stew pot or frying pan, brown the meaty sides of the short ribs in olive oil. Add the marinara sauce; cover and simmer over very low heat for 2 hours.

2. When the meat is almost falling off the bone, serve over polenta. Serve gramolata on the side as garnish.

Serves 4

Per Serving

Calories: 263
(without polenta)
GI: Zero
Carbohydrates: 5 g.
Protein: 6 g.
Fat: 28 g.

*2 tablespoons olive oil
2 pounds short ribs of beef,
    cut in 4-inch lengths
25-ounce jar tomato
    marinara sauce
Basic polenta recipe (see page
    119)
Garnish of gramolata (see
    above)*

chapter 9
International

Asian Sesame-Crusted Scallops

Sea scallops can be grilled, broiled, or sautéed. Try to get really big scallops—
called "diver" scallops. They are very sweet and velvety in texture.
These are delicious as an appetizer for four or a main course for two.

Serves 2

PER SERVING

Calories: 272
GI: Very Low
Carbohydrates: 12 g.
Protein: 27 g.
Fat: 14 g.

*2 cups Napa cabbage,
    shredded*
1 large ripe tomato, sliced
2 ounces soy sauce
1 ounce sesame oil
Juice of ½ lime
*1 inch fresh gingerroot,
    peeled and minced*
*½ pound diver scallops, each
    weighing 1+ ounce (3 to 4
    per person)*
1 egg, beaten
½ cup sesame seeds
2 tablespoons peanut oil
Salt and pepper to taste

1. Make beds on 2 serving plates with the cabbage and the tomatoes. In a small bowl, mix together the soy sauce, sesame oil, lime juice, and minced ginger to create sauce.

2. Rinse the scallops and pat them dry on paper towels. Dip scallops in beaten egg. Then cover them with sesame seeds that you have spread out on waxed paper.

3. Heat the peanut oil in a nonstick frying pan. Sear the scallops over medium heat until browned on both sides and hot through. Do not overcook, or they will get tough. Arrange the scallops over the greens and tomatoes; add salt and pepper. Drizzle with the sauce.

Indian Tandoori-Style Chicken

*Garam masala is a combination of spices used in most Indian cooking.
A basic recipe contains coriander, cinnamon, cloves, cardamom, and cumin.
Try ½ teaspoon of each as a base and then make changes to suit your taste.*

Serves 4

PER SERVING

Calories: 169
GI: Zero
Carbohydrates: 4 g.
Protein: 28 g.
Fat: 6 g.

*4 chicken breast halves,
    boneless and skinless,
    pounded thin
1 cup low-fat yogurt
1 tablespoon garam masala
2 cloves garlic, mashed*

1. In a large glass pan, marinate the chicken breasts overnight in a mixture of garam masala, garlic, and yogurt.

2. Preheat the oven or grill to 400°F. Broil or grill the chicken for 4 minutes per side. The hot oven recreates the clay oven, or tandoori, used in India to bake meats.

Asian Markets

Don't be afraid to ask the manager or owner of an Asian market about things that are unfamiliar to you. In this way, you open yourself to discovering such goodies as premade garam masala, tamarind pulp, lemongrass, and other delicious additions to your cooking.

Thai Chicken Stew with Vegetables in Coconut Cream

Asian flavorings can provide so many minimal, yet wonderful, additions to rather ordinary foods. This chicken stew is spicy and tastes very rich. It is loaded with vegetables, which reduce the GI.

Serves 4

PER SERVING

Calories: 540
GI: Low
Carbohydrates: 16 g.
Protein: 55 g.
Fat: 35 g.

2 tablespoons peanut oil
2 cloves garlic, minced
1 inch fresh gingerroot, peeled and minced
2 carrots, shredded
1 cup canned coconut cream
1 cup chicken broth
2 cups Napa cabbage, shredded
4 chicken breasts, about 5 ounces each, boneless and skinless in bite-size pieces
¼ cup soy sauce
1 teaspoon Thai chili paste (red or green) or red hot pepper sauce
2 tablespoons Asian fish sauce
1 tablespoon sesame oil
½ cup scallions, greens chopped
¼ cup cilantro, chopped

1. Sauté the garlic and ginger in the peanut oil. Add the carrots, coconut cream, and chicken broth and simmer for 10 minutes. Add the cabbage, chicken, and sauces.

2. Whisk in the chili paste. Stir in the sesame oil, scallions, and cilantro. Simmer for 20 minutes. Serve over rice.

Coconut Cream, Coconut Milk, Coconut Juice

Contrary to popular belief, coconut milk is not the liquid found inside a whole coconut (which is called coconut juice). It is made from mixing water with shredded coconut. This mixture is then squeezed through cheesecloth to filter out the coconut pieces. Coconut cream is the same as coconut milk but made with less water and more coconut.

Grilled Shrimp and Vegetables with Dipping Sauce

When you marinate shrimp, be careful not to leave it in an acidic marinade. The lime juice adds flavor, but it also will "cook" your shrimp if left too long. You can serve this over brown rice if you don't mind upping your GI.

1. Marinate shrimp for 1 hour in a mixture of lime juice, soy sauce, garlic, gingerroot, fish sauce, and peanut oil.

2. Skewer the shrimp on separate skewers from the red pepper, zucchini, and mushrooms.

3. Broil or grill the vegetables for 6 minutes, turning often. Add the shrimp and grill for about 2 minutes per side, or until shrimp turns pink.

Wooden Skewers

Wooden skewers must be presoaked to prevent them from burning. Metal skewers work fine, but they have to be washed after using, whereas you just dispose of the wooden ones.

Serves 2

PER SERVING (DIPPING SAUCE NOT INCLUDED)

Calories: 273
GI: Zero
Carbohydrates: 20 g.
Protein: 38 g.
Fat: 6 g.

---

4 wooden skewers, soaked in water for 1 hour
6 jumbo shrimp, cleaned and deveined
Juice of 1 lime
¼ cup soy sauce
2 cloves garlic, minced
1 inch gingerroot, peeled and minced
2 tablespoons Asian fish sauce
¼ cup peanut oil
1 red pepper, cored, seeded, and cut in wedges
1 medium zucchini, ends removed, cut in 1-inch pieces
6 large brown mushrooms

Skewered Chicken Sate with Baby Eggplant

This combination of grilled vegetables, chicken, and Asian flavors is delicious and complemented by the easy-to-make peanut dipping sauce.

Serves 4

PER SERVING

Calories: 438
GI: Very Low
Carbohydrates: 11 g.
Protein: 51 g.
Fat: 24 g.

12 bamboo skewers, soaked
    for 1 hour in water
1 pound skinless, boneless
    chicken breast, cut in
    bite-size chunks
2 baby eggplants, cut in
    halves lengthwise,
    unpeeled
¼ cup lemon juice
¼ cup soy sauce
Salt and pepper to taste
½ cup creamy peanut butter
¼ cup soy sauce
1 tablespoon pineapple juice
1 teaspoon chili sauce (such
    as Tabasco)
1 head romaine lettuce leaves
    (save small white hearts
    for salad)

1. Skewer the chicken and eggplants on separate skewers. Mix the lemon juice, soy sauce, salt, and pepper. Brush the lemon-soy mixture on the eggplant halves and the chicken.

2. Set grill on medium or use the broiler on high.

3. Make the peanut dipping sauce by mixing the peanut butter, soy sauce, pineapple juice, and chili sauce. If too thick, add more pineapple juice.

4. Grill the chicken and eggplants for 4 to 5 minutes per side, turning frequently.

5. Dip skewered chicken and eggplant in peanut dipping sauce and enjoy! Use the lettuce leaves as wraps to prevent burning your hands or getting sticky.

Filet Mignon Strips with Exotic Mushrooms

This dish gives you both fat and protein with the steak.
To add important veggies and fiber, check out the suggested sauces.

1. In a hot, nonstick pan, melt 1 teaspoon butter over medium-high flame. Sprinkle the steak strips with salt and pepper.

2. Sauté the filet mignon to desired doneness, about 1 minute per side for rare to medium. Remove the filet mignon strips to warm plates.

3. Using the pan in which you sautéed the filet mignon, sauté mushrooms with 1 teaspoon butter until softened.

4. Add the beef broth to the pan and reduce heat. Simmer for 2 minutes; add brandy or cognac and peppercorns, stirring to get any brown bits off the pan. Pour Fresh Tomato Sauce for Steak or Chicken (see page 134) over the filet mignon. Add Sour Cream Chive Sauce (see page 136) if desired.

> ❤ *Substitute olive oil for butter in this recipe to* ❤
> *reduce the amount of calories and fat.*

PER SERVING

Calories: 359
GI: Zero
Carbohydrates: 0 g.
Protein: 44 g.
Fat: 11 g.

2 teaspoons butter
Salt and pepper to taste
⅔ pound filet mignon, cut in strips
6 shitake mushrooms, trimmed and chopped
¼ cup beef broth
2 tablespoons brandy or cognac
1 tablespoon green peppercorns

Fresh Tomato Sauce for Steak or Chicken

This is a very versatile sauce—use it on any meat or poultry.

Blanch the tomatoes in boiling water, drain, slip off skins, and chop. In a small bowl, mix the chopped tomatoes with the rest of the ingredients. Serve warm.

Long Noodles for Chinese New Year

Every dish at a Chinese New Year's party has meaning. The long noodles represent long life! You can find these noodles at Asian markets and some supermarkets.

1. To make the sauce, begin by heating the sesame oil. Stir in the garlic, scallions, and water chestnuts, and sauté for a few minutes. Add the almonds, sugar, sherry, and soy sauce. Mix well and set aside in a large bowl.

2. Cook noodles to package directions. Drain and mix into the sauce. Serve hot or at room temperature.

Tofu with Shrimp and Vegetables

Almost any dish can be pepped up with hot pepper sauce, lemon zest, lemon or lime juice, or aromatic herbs. Try making any basic sauce and throw in any of these. Keep tasting until you get more zip! This is a basic stir-fry with a kick.

Heat oil in a wok or nonstick pan over medium-high heat. Stir in the ginger, bean sprouts, and snap peas. Stir and cook for 2 minutes. Add the rest of the ingredients, stirring until shrimp turns pink. Serve immediately.

Types of Tofu

Tofu is a versatile food that comes in a few different types, all of which are low in calories and high in protein. Firm tofu is best for grilling, whereas soft tofu is suitable for blended dishes or soups. Satin or silken tofu is more creamy and custard-like but does come in extra-firm varieties that you can stir-fry.

Serves 2

PER SERVING

Calories: 270
GI: Zero
Carbohydrates: 14 g.
Protein: 29 g.
Fat: 13 g.

2 teaspoons peanut oil
1 teaspoon Asian sesame oil
1 teaspoon fresh gingerroot, peeled and minced
1 cup bean sprouts
1 cup sugar snap peas
1 teaspoon tahini
4 ounces satin tofu
6 ounces small shrimp, peeled and deveined
1 tablespoon soy sauce
1 teaspoon Thai chili paste, or red hot pepper sauce

Sour Cream Chive Sauce

This is a rich and creamy spicy sauce.

Mix all ingredients in a small bowl; serve chilled.

> *You can replace the sour cream in this sauce
> with low-fat sour cream.*

Makes ½ cup, serves 4

PER SERVING

Calories: 62
GI: Zero
Carbohydrates: 2cg.
Protein: 0g.
Fat: 6 g.

½ cup sour cream
¼ cup chives, snipped fine
  with kitchen shears
1 teaspoon prepared
  horseradish, or to taste
Salt and pepper to taste

Moroccan Couscous with Harissa and Artichoke Hearts

This can be served hot or cold, as a side dish or as a lunch.
Harissa is a hot red chili paste that comes in tubes from specialty markets.
If you are unable to find Harissa, you can use red hot sauce.

1. Thaw artichokes and boil for 10 minutes in water to cover.

2. Sauté the garlic and onion in olive oil until soft, about 8 minutes.

3. Bring 1-½ cups of water to a boil and add couscous, stirring. When water is absorbed, add harissa, salt, pepper, and vegetables. Serve hot or cold.

Serves 4

PER SERVING

Calories: 302
GI: Very Low
Carbohydrates: 57 g.
Protein: 10 g.
Fat: 5 g.

1 tablespoon olive oil
2 cloves garlic, chopped
1 small red onion, chopped
10-ounce box frozen
  artichoke hearts
1-½ cups water
1 cup couscous
1 teaspoon harissa
Salt and pepper to taste

Curried Lamb

Shoulder lamb chops work best for this inexpensive dish. Remember that when buying meat on the bone for a recipe that you have to allow for the weight of the bones. The bones add a great deal of flavor to stews and soups, even though you have to take them out later.

1. Heat the canola oil over medium flame in a large pot. Brown the lamb and then add the rest of the vegetables.

2. Stir in the chicken broth. Mix the curry powder with the white wine to dissolve it and stir into the pot.

3. Cover the pot and reduce heat to a simmer. Cook over very low heat for 3 hours. Cool and remove the bones and any fat that has come to the top of the stew.

4. Reheat just before serving.

Serves 4

PER SERVING

Calories: 420
GI: Zero
Carbohydrates: 22 g.
Protein: 37 g.
Fat: 19 g.

2 tablespoons canola oil
2 pounds shoulder lamb
  chops, bone in, trimmed
  of fat
4 white onions, chopped
4 cloves garlic, chopped
2 serrano or Scotch bonnet
  chilies, cored, seeded, and
  chopped
1 inch gingerroot, peeled and
  minced
2 carrots, peeled and
  chopped
1 stalk celery with leaves,
  chopped
2 fresh tomatoes, chopped
1 red roasted pepper,
  chopped
1 cup chicken broth
½ cup dry white wine
2 tablespoons curry powder
Salt and pepper to taste

Moroccan Couscous with Apricots

*Couscous is very small pasta, popular in Morocco and
other areas of the Middle East. It cooks quickly and lends itself
to many dishes and is a good substitute for rice.*

Serves 4

PER SERVING

Calories: 328
GI: Very Low
Carbohydrates: 67 g.
Protein: 8 g.
Fat: 4 g.

*8 ounces dried apricots
1 tablespoon sugar
Juice and rind of ½ lemon
1-½ cups boiling water
1 teaspoon salt, or to taste
1 cup couscous
½ teaspoon coriander seeds,
    ground
1 teaspoon dried sage
    leaves, crumbled, or 1
    tablespoon fresh sage,
    torn
1 tablespoon butter*

1. Cut the apricots in quarters and soak in 2 cups hot water with sugar for 1 hour.

2. Stir the couscous into the boiling water. Add apricots, lemon juice, and lemon rind.

3. Cook, stirring, until water has absorbed. Add coriander and sage.

4. Stir in butter. Serve hot or warm.

> *In this couscous recipe, you can substitute olive oil or
> heart-healthy margarine for butter.*

Couscous Variety

Couscous is unique because it is equally delicious with both fruits and vegetables, working well as a sweet or savory dish or even as a sweet-savory dish.

Eggplant Soufflé

Smooth and creamy in texture, this is an Indian favorite.
Often, the eggplant is simply puréed and spiced—this is more of a fusion dish.

1. Wrap the eggplant in aluminum foil packages with 1 teaspoon water added to each. Roast the eggplant at 400°F for 1 hour, or until very soft when pricked with a fork. Cool, cut in half, scoop out flesh, and discard skin.

2. Heat peanut oil and sauté garlic and onion over medium heat until softened, about 8 to 10 minutes. Mix with eggplant and purée in the food processor or blender until very smooth. Mix in egg yolks and pulse, adding salt, pepper, and curry powder. Place in a 1-quart soufflé dish, prepared with nonstick spray.

3. Preheat oven to 400°F. Beat the egg whites until stiff. Fold into the eggplant mixture. Bake until puffed and golden, about 45 minutes.

Serves 4

PER SERVING

Calories: 126
GI: Low
Carbohydrates: 13 g.
Protein: 9 g.
Fat: 9 g.

1 large or 2 medium
*   eggplants*
1 tablespoon peanut oil
2 cloves garlic, minced
1 small white onion, minced
4 eggs, separated
Salt and pepper to taste
1 teaspoon curry powder,
*   or to taste*
Nonstick spray

Saffron Rice

Saffron is the most expensive spice in the world.
It adds a lovely golden color to rice, breads, and pasta.

Serves 4

PER SERVING

Calories: 107
GI: Very Low
Carbohydrates: 57 g.
Protein: 8 g.
Fat: 5 g.

½ cup white onion, chopped
1 tablespoon butter
½ teaspoon saffron
1 cup basmati rice
2-½ cups chicken broth
Salt and pepper to taste

1. Sauté the onion for 8 minutes in butter in a large saucepan. Blend in the saffron and add rice, mixing to coat.

2. Add the chicken broth, salt, and pepper. Reduce heat to a simmer. Cover and cook rice for 30 minutes or until it has absorbed liquid and fluffs nicely with a fork.

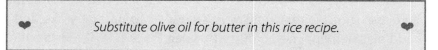

Substitute olive oil for butter in this rice recipe.

Hawaiian Fresh Ham, Roasted with Pineapple and Rum

Fresh ham is basically leg of pork. It is a tender
white meat and a great fall or winter dish.

Serves 10

PER SERVING

Calories: 608
GI: Low
Carbohydrates: 27 g.
Protein: 28 g.
Fat: 37 g.

2 cups pineapple juice
1 cup rum
¼ cup brown sugar, or to taste
½ teaspoon cloves, ground
Salt and hot red pepper sauce
    to taste
6 pounds fresh ham, some fat
    (about ¼ inch)
1 fresh pineapple, peeled and
    cut in chunks

1. Preheat oven to 350°F. Reduce the pineapple juice to 1 cup over high heat. Add rum, brown sugar, cloves, salt, and red pepper sauce.

2. Score the fat left on the ham with a sharp knife and place ham in a roasting pan. Baste with pineapple syrup. Roast and baste for 3 hours, basting often. If the bottom of the pan starts to burn, add water.

3. Surround with the fresh pineapple chunks in the last hour of cooking. If the ham gets too brown, tent with aluminum foil.

4. Serve with the pan drippings on the side and caramelized pineapple chunks, also on the side.

Nova Scotia Mussels in Herbed Cream Sauce

*Farm-raised mussels are wonderful—no sand, no beards,
and shipped all over the country as soon as they are harvested.*

1. Scrub mussels and make sure they are tightly closed. Tap together and listen for a sharp clicking sound to make sure they are fresh. Place them in a pot with the wine and shallots. Bring to a boil over high heat.

2. As the mussels open, remove them to a large bowl. Discard any mussels that do not open. Reduce heat and add herbs, heavy cream, and pepper.

3. Remove the top shell from each mussel, return to the pot. Reheat and serve.

Farm-Raised Shellfish

Farm-raised mussels are not only easier for you to prepare, but they are also an environmentally friendly choice. Shellfish are often raised in bags suspended over the seafloor. They filter small organisms out of the water, improving water quality, and harvesting them does not disrupt the ecosystem.

Serves 2

PER SERVING

Calories: 189
GI: Very Low
Carbohydrates: 5 g.
Protein: 8 g.
Fat: 14 g.

*1 pound mussels
¼ cup dry white wine
2 shallots, minced
½ teaspoon thyme, dried,
    or 1 teaspoon fresh
10 fresh basil leaves, torn
¼ cup heavy cream
½ cup fresh parsley, chopped
Freshly ground black pepper
    to taste*

Jasmine Rice with Rosewater

Jasmine-flavored rice and rosewater are available at Asian markets.

Bring the water and rosewater to a boil. Add the rice, salt, and pepper. Reduce heat to a simmer; stir in salt and pepper. Cover and cook for 30 minutes or to package directions.

Serves 4

PER SERVING

Calories: 56
GI: Low
Carbohydrates: 43 g.
Protein: 7 g.
Fat: 1 g.

¼ cup rosewater
2 cups water
1 cup jasmine rice
Salt and pepper to taste

Chicken Française with Fine Herbs and Red Grapes

This French classic is highly adaptable. This version is innovative without losing the delicious sweetness of the chicken and tang of the lemon.

1. Pound the chicken until flattened to ½ inch in thickness. Dip it in the egg and then in a mixture of salt, pepper, flour, chives, and rosemary. Coat thoroughly.

2. Heat the olive oil over medium flame. Sauté the chicken until golden on both sides. Remove to a warm platter.

3. Add the lemon juice, chicken broth, and grapes to the pan. Bring to a boil. Return the chicken to the pan to finish cooking. Pour the sauce over the chicken and serve on warm plates.

Serves 2

PER SERVING

Calories: 287
GI: Very Low
Carbohydrates: 48 g.
Protein: 4 g.
Fat: 11 g.

⅔ pound chicken breasts,
    boneless and skinless
1 egg, well beaten
Salt and pepper to taste
2 tablespoons flour
2 teaspoons chives, snipped
1 teaspoon rosemary leaves,
    finely minced
1 tablespoon olive oil
Juice of ½ lemon
¼ cup chicken broth
10 red grapes, halved

chapter 10
Vegetarian

Stuffed Artichokes

These can be prepared in advance and then heated up just before serving. Artichoke hearts are wonderful in salads, and the individual leaves are delicious dipped in hot butter or Hollandaise sauce and the meat scraped off with your teeth. Remember to remove the choke—it is indigestible and spiny.

**Serves 4
(1 large or 2 medium
artichokes per person)**

Per Serving

Calories: 238
GI: Very Low
Carbohydrates: 29 g.
Protein: 5 g.
Fat: 13 g.

4 large artichokes
Juice and rind of ½ lemon
1 teaspoon coriander seeds
2 tablespoons butter or olive
   oil
1 celery stalk, chopped
¼ cup Vidalia onion, chopped
2 cloves garlic, chopped
1 cup corn bread crumbs or
   commercial corn bread
   stuffing
1 teaspoon oregano
Salt and pepper to taste
⅔ cup vegetable broth to
   moisten crumbs
4 tablespoons Parmesan
   cheese (4 teaspoons
   reserved for topping)
4 teaspoons butter or olive oil
   for topping
Nonstick spray

1. Using scissors, remove the sharp leaf points of the artichokes and cut off the ends of the stems. Pull off the large outside leaves. Bring 2 quarts of water to a boil with the lemon and coriander over high heat. Add the artichokes and return to a boil. Reduce to a simmer and cook artichokes for 15 minutes. Drain and let cool.

2. Heat the butter or olive oil and add the celery, onion, and garlic. Sauté over medium heat for 10 minutes, or until softened. Add the corn bread crumbs, oregano, salt and pepper, broth, and part of the cheese.

3. Cut the artichokes in halves and remove the "chokes." Arrange in a baking dish prepared with nonstick spray. Spoon the stuffing into the areas left by the chokes.

4. Sprinkle with cheese and dot with extra butter or drizzle with olive oil. At this point, the stuffed artichokes can be covered and refrigerated. When ready to bake, remove wrapping and bake for 30 minutes at 350°F.

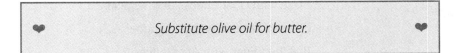

Substitute olive oil for butter.

Cheese Soufflé

Aside from the cheese you might buy for this, it's also a wonderful way to use up bits of cheese that are in your fridge, left over from a dinner party, and so forth. Plus, cheese soufflé is really an excellent dish for lunch or supper.

1. Preheat the oven to 375°F. Prepare two, 2-cup individual soufflé dishes by buttering the insides. Then, sprinkle the Parmesan cheese around the bottom and up the sides.

2. Melt the rest of the butter and mix in the shallots. Cook for 3 minutes and stir in the flour and seasonings. Cook and stir until well blended. Whisk in the warm milk. Continue to whisk and stir until very thick.

3. Remove from heat and stir in the cheese. Beat the egg yolks and add 1 tablespoon of the hot cheese mixture to the yolks and then whisk in the rest. Fold in the beaten egg whites. Pour into the dishes.

4. Bake for 20 minutes or until brown and puffed. Serve immediately.

> Substitute nonfat milk for 2% milk and replace butter with olive oil. ♥

Serves 2

PER SERVING

Calories: 580
GI: Very Low
Carbohydrates: 8 g.
Protein: 40 g.
Fat: 42 g.

¼ cup Parmesan cheese
1 teaspoon butter
2 shallots, minced
1 tablespoon flour
Salt and pepper to taste
⅛ teaspoon nutmeg
⅛ teaspoon cayenne pepper
½ cup 2% milk, warmed
¾ cup Cheddar cheese, grated (you may substitute or add, blue, Gorgonzola, or Gruyere)
3 egg yolks
4 egg whites, beaten stiff

Cheese Fondue with Crudités

This is an interactive party dish. Use fresh, raw vegetables such as broccoli, cauliflower, peppers, zucchini, onion wedges, or whatever you like! You can poach the broccoli and cauliflower for easy chewing. Kirsch is a German wine made from cherries.

Serves 2

PER SERVING

Calories: 537
GI: Zero
Carbohydrates: 5 g.
Protein: 24 g.
Fat: 36 g.

1 clove garlic
⅔ cup dry white wine
½ pound Gruyere cheese, grated
1 tablespoon Kirsch
⅛ teaspoon nutmeg
Salt and pepper to taste
A variety of your favorite veggies

1. Mash the garlic to a paste. In a chafing dish or large flame-proof casserole, heat the wine and blend in the garlic.

2. Add the cheese, a handful at a time, stirring constantly. When all of the cheese is melted, stir in the Kirsch, nutmeg, salt, and pepper.

3. Using individual skewers, spear a piece of vegetable, dip in the fondue, and enjoy!

Clam Soup

This is best with fresh clams and bottled clam juice. The fresh clams in the shell make for a lovely presentation.

Serves 2

PER SERVING

Calories: 292
GI: Very Low
Carbohydrates: 32 g.
Protein: 14 g.
Fat: 13 g.

1 teaspoon butter
½ cup sweet onion, chopped
½ cup potato, peeled and chopped
1 stalk celery with leaves, chopped
1-½ cups clam broth
12 littleneck clams, scrubbed
Pepper to taste
¼ cup light cream
2 sprigs parsley

1. Melt the butter over medium heat and sauté the onion until soft. Add potatoes, celery, and clam broth. Cover, reduce heat, and simmer until the potatoes are soft, about 15 minutes.

2. Drop in the clams, and as soon as they open, add pepper and light cream. Garnish with parsley. Serve immediately.

> *Replace butter with olive oil.*

Mini Veggie Burgers

These are quite good and easy to make.

1. Pulse all but the rice and canola oil in the food processor or blender. Turn into a bowl.

2. Add brown rice to bean mixture.

3. Form into mini burgers. Heat oil to 300°F and fry burgers until very hot. Serve on rolls or plain.

The Praises of Brown Rice

Unlike white rice, which is rice with its outer layers removed, brown rice has lost only the hard outer hull of the grain when it gets to the store. As a result, brown rice contains many more nutrients than its more processed relative. Also, the fiber in brown rice decreases your risk for colon cancer and helps lower cholesterol!

Serves 4

PER SERVING

Calories: 251
GI: Very Low
Carbohydrates: 34 g.
Protein: 11 g.
Fat: 10 g.

13-ounce can red kidney beans, drained
½ cup dried bread crumbs (more if beans are very wet)
½ cup red onion, chopped
2 tablespoons Worcestershire sauce
2 tablespoons barbecue sauce
1 egg
1 teaspoon oregano, rosemary, thyme, basil, or sage
Salt and pepper to taste
½ cup brown rice, cooked
2 tablespoons canola oil

Black Bean Casserole

*Vegetarians may find themselves running low on protein.
Cheese, whether low-fat (like Parmesan) or high-fat (like Brie), adds flavor
and will supply needed calcium and protein. This casserole provides protein in
cheese and beans and is hearty at a cookout or as a supper.*

Serves 6

PER SERVING

Calories: 449
GI: Very Low
Carbohydrates: 41 g.
Protein: 18 g.
Fat: 25 g.

2 tablespoons olive oil
1 medium red onion,
   chopped
2 cloves garlic, minced
2 red or yellow peppers,
   cored, seeded, and
   chopped
4 tomatillos, peeled and
   chopped
4 ripe Roma or plum
   tomatoes, chopped
2 13-ounce cans black beans,
   drained
Salt and pepper to taste
½ pound Monterey Jack
   or pepper jack cheese,
   grated, ⅔ cup set aside
   for topping
1 cup sour cream
¼ cup chili sauce
1 cup bread crumbs for
   topping
1 teaspoon oregano

1. Using an ovenproof casserole dish, heat the olive oil over medium heat and add onion, garlic, peppers, and tomatillos. After they have softened, add tomatoes. Cover and simmer for 10 minutes.

2. Stir in 1 can of the beans; sprinkle with salt, pepper, and half the cheese, mixing well.

3. Mix the sour cream and chili sauce. Mix with the other can of beans; sprinkle with more salt and pepper. Spoon mixture over the casserole. Make the topping by mixing the remaining cheese with bread crumbs and oregano.

4. Bake in a 350°F oven for 25 minutes or until the topping is browned and the beans are hot. When serving, dig the spoon deeply to get all of the flavors!

❤ *Substitute low-fat sour cream for regular sour cream.* ❤

Stuffed Peppers with Rice and Spice

Green peppers are divine, but red, yellow, and orange peppers have more vitamin C. You can mix leftover veggies in with the rice or lentils for an impromptu supper. This one is a favorite for a midwinter lunch.

1. Heat olive oil over medium-low flame. Stir in onions and garlic and sauté for 4 minutes. Add the parsley, coriander, Tabasco, thyme, salt, and pepper. When well mixed, spoon in the rice, stirring to coat with oil, herbs, and spices.

2. Preheat the oven to 350°F. Split the peppers lengthwise and lay them in a baking pan prepared with nonstick spray. Fill the peppers with the rice mixture.

3. Pour the pureed tomatoes over the top. Sprinkle with Parmesan cheese. Bake for 35 minutes.

Serves 2

PER SERVING

Calories: 329
GI: Very Low
Carbohydrates: 41 g.
Protein: 9 g.
Fat: 16 g.

1 ounce olive oil
¼ cup red onion, chopped fine
1 clove garlic, minced
2 sprigs fresh parsley, minced
1 teaspoon coriander seeds, cracked
Tabasco sauce to taste
1 teaspoon dried thyme
Salt and pepper to taste
1 cup basmati rice, cooked
2 extra large sweet red or green bell peppers
2 cups plum tomatoes, drained and puréed
2 tablespoons Parmesan cheese, grated
Nonstick spray

Smoked Salmon, Eggs, and Cheese Puffed Casserole

This is an excellent brunch dish. Serve with a salad on the side and feast!

Serves 2

PER SERVING

Calories: 478
GI: Low
Carbohydrates: 20 g.
Protein: 27 g.
Fat: 33 g.

4 eggs, separated
4 ounces cream cheese, at
room temperature
⅛ pound smoked salmon
½ cup white onion, chopped
Pepper to taste
2 slices whole grain bread
¼ cup 2% milk
Nonstick spray

1. Preheat the oven to 400°F. Beat the egg whites until stiff and set aside. Cut bread into quarters.

2. Place the egg yolks, cream cheese, onion, pepper, bread, and milk in the food processor or blender and purée until smooth and creamy.

3. Prepare a 1-quart soufflé dish with nonstick spray; place bread in the bottom of the dish. In a bowl, fold the beaten egg whites into the cheese mixture and gently mix in the salmon. Pour into the dish.

4. Bake for 30 minutes or until puffed and golden.

> *Substitute nonfat milk for 2% milk and*
> *replace sour cream with low-fat sour cream.*

Omega-3 Fatty Acids

Salmon is an excellent source of omega-3 fatty acids, which can improve heart function and lower blood pressure. You can get omega-3 fatty acids from most cold-water fish, such as albacore tuna, salmon, and trout, which tend to have more of these good fats than other fish.

Ratatouille with White Beans

*This is a classic French dish of stewed vegetables,
often including tomatoes and eggplant, served as an appetizer or side dish.
Serving it over beans makes it a bit heartier and very satisfying.*

1. Heat the olive oil. Sauté the eggplant, onion, garlic, and zucchini for 5 minutes.

2. Add tomatoes, herbs, salt, and pepper. Cover and simmer for 10 minutes. Warm the beans and serve by pouring vegetables over the beans.

A Provencal Delight

Ratatouille is a versatile vegetable stew that can be served hot (either alone or as a side dish), room temperature, or even cold as an appetizer on toast or crackers. As an appetizer, it is similar to the Italian tomato, onion, and basil salad called bruschetta.

Serves 2

PER SERVING

Calories: 409
GI: Very Low
Carbohydrates: 59 g.
Protein: 24 g.
Fat: 16 g.

¼ cup olive oil
2 baby eggplants, chopped
1 onion, sliced
2 cloves garlic, minced
1 small zucchini, chopped
*2 medium tomatoes,
    chopped*
*1 teaspoon each of dried
    parsley, thyme, and
    rosemary; if fresh, 1
    tablespoon of each*
Salt and pepper to taste
1 13-ounce can white beans

Okra Stuffed with Green Peppercorns

This is a delightful Indian dish. You can make it in advance and warm it up later. It's a spicy side dish when you are serving rice or curry, and okra is a nice vegetable alternative if you get sick of the usual broccoli, asparagus, and zucchini.

1. Poach the okra in the vegetable broth until slightly softened, about 4 minutes. Remove from the broth and place on a work surface, reserving broth in the saucepan.

2. Rinse the peppercorns and poke them into and down the center of the okra. Return to broth; add butter and cumin. Add salt and pepper to taste. Serve as is or with rice.

> *Replace butter with olive oil or heart-healthy margarine.*

Cold Tomato Soup with Tofu

Tofu is an excellent meat substitute. It's light and filling and absorbs other flavors in a dish. You can blend it and use it instead of yogurt or cream for a creamy look and texture.
This is a perfect vegan lunch that you can serve hot or cold.

Place all ingredients in the blender and purée until smooth.

Broccoli Rabe with Lemon and Cheese

Broccoli rabe is somewhat bitter and has a real snap to the flavor. It is wonderful when prepoached in boiling water and then sautéed in oil with a bit of garlic and lemon juice. Serve this recipe over rice, pasta, or on its own.

1. Bring the water to a boil; add salt and broccoli rabe. Reduce heat and simmer for 6 to 8 minutes. Drain and shock under cold water and dry on paper towels.

2. Heat olive oil over medium-low heat and sauté the garlic for 5 minutes. Cut the broccoli rabe stems in 2-inch pieces and add to the garlic and olive oil. Sprinkle with lemon juice, salt, and pepper. Serve the Parmesan cheese at the table.

Serves 4

PER SERVING

Calories: 81
GI: Zero
Carbohydrates: 2 g.
Protein: 2 g.
Fat: 8 g.

1 quart water
1 teaspoon salt
½ cup loosely packed broccoli rabe, ends trimmed
2 tablespoons olive oil
2 cloves garlic, chopped
1 tablespoon lemon juice
Salt and pepper to taste
2 tablespoons Parmesan cheese

Wild Rice with Walnuts and Apples

This is a wonderful side dish and very filling.

While the rice is cooking, sauté the shallots and apple in the olive oil over medium heat for 5 minutes. Just before serving, mix all ingredients together.

Serves 4

PER SERVING

Calories: 417
GI: Very Low
Carbohydrates: 31 g.
Protein: 8 g.
Fat: 32 g.

2 cups wild rice, cooked to package directions
¼ cup olive oil
2 shallots
1 tart apple, peeled, cored, and chopped
½ cup walnuts, toasted
Salt and pepper to taste

Grilled Peaches Filled with Mascarpone Cheese and Rosemary

Serves 2

PER SERVING

Calories: 61
GI: Very Low
Carbohydrates: 7 g.
Protein: 46 g.
Fat: 3 g.

2 ripe peaches, split, pits
  removed
4 teaspoons mascarpone
  cheese, at room
  temperature
1 teaspoon fresh rosemary,
  chopped
Salt and pepper to taste

*You may serve this as a savory brunch dish,
or mix the mascarpone with some sugar for a dessert.*

Place the peaches cut side down on a hot grill until they soften, about 4 minutes. Mix the cheese, rosemary, salt, and pepper. Turn peaches and stuff. Grill for 2 to 3 minutes.

Pizza with Goat Cheese and Vegetables

8 slices

PER SERVING (PER SLICE)

Calories: 178
GI: Low
Carbohydrates: 9 g.
Protein: 6 g.
Fat: 13 g.

1 pound pizza dough
1 cup tomato sauce from a jar
  or your own
1 medium zucchini, sliced
  thinly
1 small onion, cut thinly
20 Greek or Italian olives,
  pitted and sliced
2 teaspoons olive oil
8 ounces goat cheese

*You can buy pizza dough from almost any supermarket, bakery, or pizza
parlor. When you top the pizza with a good quality sauce, extra veggies,
and goat cheese, you have a marvelous lunch or supper.*

1. Preheat oven to 475°F. Roll out the pizza dough to fit a 12-inch pan or pizza stone. Spread with sauce. Arrange the zucchini over the sauce.

2. Sprinkle with onion and olives and spray with olive oil. Dot the top with cheese and bake for 15 minutes, or until the crust is brown, the cheese melts, and the topping bubbles.

Planked Salmon with Dill Sauce

This is a very festive and delicious way to prepare salmon. The use of a cedar plank and juniper berries are reminiscent of Native American cooking.

1. Soak the plank in water. When thoroughly soaked, lightly oil the side on which the salmon will lay. Set the salmon on the plank. Sprinkle with lemon juice and press the juniper berries into the flesh at intervals. Add salt, pepper, and lemon slices.

2. Place the plank over indirect heat on a hot grill and close lid. Roast for about 15 to 20 minutes or until the salmon begins to flake.

3. Mix the rest of the ingredients together in a small bowl and serve with the fish.

> *In this recipe, you can substitute low-fat mayonnaise for regular mayonnaise.*

Fish Bones

The larger the fish, the more likely you will find bones in a filet. Before cooking, hold a pair of pliers and run the finger of your other hand down the filet, against the grain. Whenever you feel a bone, press down close to it. It will pop up, and you can then pull it out with the pliers.

Serves 10

PER SERVING

Calories: 388
GI: Zero
Carbohydrates: 2 g.
Protein: 32 g.
Fat: 28 g.

---

1 cedar plank (available at specialty cooking stores)
Grapeseed oil
3-½ pounds salmon filet, checked for pin bones
Juice of 1 lemon
8 juniper berries
Salt and pepper to taste
1 lemon, thinly sliced
1 cup mayonnaise
¼ cup fresh dill weed, chopped
1 teaspoon horseradish
Salt and pepper to taste

Poached Eggs with Asparagus and Hollandaise Sauce

This makes a festive, holiday breakfast, brunch, or late supper.

Serves 4

PER SERVING

Calories: 538
GI: Very Low to Low
Carbohydrates: 33 g.
Protein: 24 g.
Fat: 37 g.

1 pound bunch of asparagus, ends trimmed, blanched in boiling water
4 English muffins, toasted
10 eggs
Juice of ½ lemon
¼ pound unsalted butter, melted
⅛ teaspoon cayenne pepper
1 tablespoon vinegar
Salt and pepper to taste

1. Set the blanched asparagus on a warmed plate and reserve. Place 2 eggs and lemon juice in the blender. On low speed, add the melted butter and cayenne pepper. Return to pan to rewarm over low heat, stirring often.

2. Poach the remaining 8 eggs in boiling water to which the vinegar has been added. Make individual plates with a toasted muffin, a spoonful of sauce, asparagus, 2 eggs, and more sauce. Sprinkle with salt and pepper.

> ♥ *Substitute olive oil or heart-healthy margarine for butter in this recipe.* ♥

Pumpkin Risotto

*This is a fine main course or a side dish,
depending on what else you are serving.*

1. Peel pumpkin and remove the seeds. Dice pumpkin to make 2 cups. Melt the butter or margarine in a large flameproof casserole over medium heat. Add the rice and stir to coat. Mix in the pumpkin.

2. Stirring constantly, slowly pour ½ cup of the broth into the rice mixture. Stirring, add the cloves, sage, salt, and pepper.

3. When the rice has absorbed the broth, the pot will hiss. Continue to add broth a little at a time until the rice has absorbed all of it. If still dry, add water, as with the broth, a little at a time.

4. Serve hot or at room temperature.

Rice Texture

The rice you use in risotto should give the dish a creamy texture, but be careful not to overcook—there should also be a firmness to the inside part of the grain of rice.

Serves 4

PER SERVING

Calories: 116
GI: Low
Carbohydrates: 24 g.
Protein: 2 g.
Fat: 3 g.

*1 small pumpkin (about
3 pounds)
1 tablespoon butter or
margarine
1 cup basmati rice
4 cups vegetable broth
⅛ teaspoon cloves, ground
1 teaspoon sage, dried, or
4 fresh sage leaves, torn
Salt and pepper to taste*

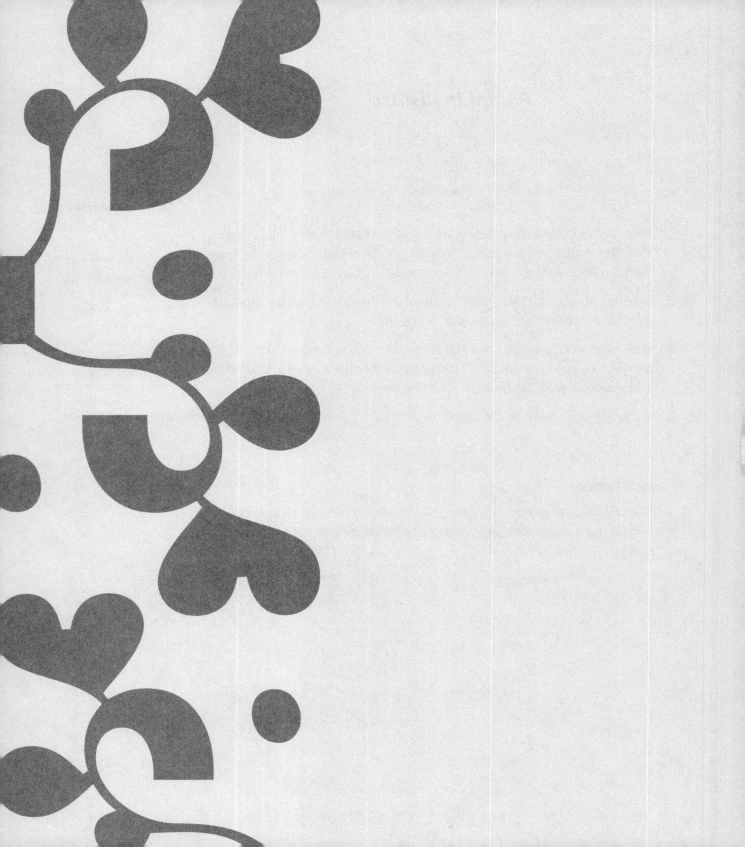

chapter 11
Energizing Meals and Sides

Sirloin Steak and Tomato Salad on Scandinavian Flat Bread

*Scandinavian flat bread, which you can find at most supermarkets,
makes a wonderful, crunchy base for lots of good things to eat.
It's flavored with rye and can support strong flavors.*

1. Marinate the steak in French dressing for 20 minutes. Sprinkle with salt and pepper. Heat a frying pan to medium high and use nonstick spray or oil.

2. Quickly sear the slices of steak on both sides and pile on the flat bread. Add tomato slices and a bit more French dressing. Serve and crunch away!

Mushroom and Cheese Salad

*When you are in a hurry and need a lot of zip,
both in your taste buds and your body, try this!*

1. Whisk the French dressing and egg together with the Parmesan cheese.

2. Brush the mushrooms clean and thinly slice.

3. Arrange the salad greens on a chilled plate. Add the cheese, mushrooms, and capers. Sprinkle with dressing. Garnish to taste.

London Broil with Onions and Sweet Potato Sticks

This will give you a real energy boost! To get the maximum energy out of this recipe, eat slowly and enjoy a smaller portion.

1. Heat olive oil over medium flame in a frying pan. Season the steak with salt, pepper, and steak seasoning. Add steak and onions to the pan and sauté until the steak reaches the desired level of doneness.

2. Sprinkle steak with hot pepper flakes and Worcestershire sauce. Mix in salsa and stuff the red peppers with the mixture.

3. Serve with the baked sweet potato sticks on the side.

What Is London Broil?

Surprisingly, London broil is not actually a cut of beef but is, in fact, a cooking method. Although many grocery stores and butchers may have a very lean piece of meat labeled as a London broil, it is likely to be a top round roast or top round steak.

Serves 2

PER SERVING

Calories: 384
(with baked sweet potato sticks)
GI: Moderate
Carbohydrates: 26 g.
Protein: 38 g.
Fat: 15 g.

1 tablespoon olive oil
½ pound London broil, diced
Salt and pepper
Steak seasoning
½ cup sweet onion, chopped
Hot red pepper flakes to taste
1 teaspoon Worcestershire
    sauce
2 tablespoons salsa
2 large sweet red bell
    peppers, cut lengthwise,
    cored and seeded
Baked Sweet Potato Sticks
    (see page 165)

Poached Chicken Breasts with Grapes and Noodles

PER SERVING

Calories: 332
GI: Low
Carbohydrates: 24 g.
Protein: 42 g.
Fat: 10 g.

½ Vidalia onion, chopped
2 cloves garlic, chopped
1 tablespoon butter or oil
2 ¼ pound chicken breasts,
    boneless and skinless
Dusting of flour
Salt and pepper to taste
½ cup apple juice or cider
Juice of ½ lime
1 cup green or red seedless
    grapes
½ pound of your favorite
    noodles

Carbohydrates can give you a lift and keep you going if they are slow-release material. Sugary carbohydrates give you a quick lift and then your energy drops off. A bit of sugar is okay when you know you will be burning it off. You also need protein for energy and endurance.

1. Sauté the onions and garlic in the butter or oil. Dust the chicken breasts with flour and sprinkle with salt and pepper. Sear in the pan with the garlic and onions.

2. Add the apple juice or cider, lime juice, and grapes.

3. Cook noodles according to package directions.

4. Cover and simmer for 10 minutes. Serve over noodles.

Chicken Breasts with Orange Glaze and Oranges

This is an excellent way to cook chicken.
The flavors complement each other and make a delicious meal.

1. Mix the first seven ingredients. Paint on the chicken.

2. Roast the chicken in a 350°F oven, surrounded by orange slices, for 35 minutes. Serve over rice.

Serves 2

Per Serving (excluding rice)

Calories: 225
GI: Low
Carbohydrates: 26 g.
Protein: 22 g.
Fat: 6 g.

2 tablespoons marmalade
2 tablespoons orange juice
1 tablespoon soy sauce
1 teaspoon hot pepper sauce
1 teaspoon thyme leaves, dried
1 teaspoon cardamom, ground
1 tablespoon sesame oil
½ pound chicken breast, halved, bone in, skin removed
1 orange, sliced thinly, skin on
1-½ cups cooked brown rice

Celeriac Slaw for Garnish or Appetizers

In France, celeriac (a vegetable in the celery family) is used at cocktail time
on a toasted piece of baguette, dressed with a shrimp, a mussel,
or some other delicious treat. You can put this slaw next to most meat,
fish, or poultry for a delicious counterpoint.

Place the celeriac in a bowl. In a separate bowl, mix the mayonnaise, vinegar, thyme, salt, pepper, and mustard. Pour over the celeriac and serve as a garnish or as part of an appetizer tray.

Makes ⅔ cup, 6 servings

Per Serving

Calories: 45
GI: Zero
Carbohydrates: 9 g.
Protein: 1 g.
Fat: 1 g.

1 celeriac bulb, peeled and grated coarsely
1 tablespoon low-fat mayonnaise
1 tablespoon white wine vinegar
Pinch dried thyme
Salt and pepper to taste
1 teaspoon dry English mustard

Chicken Scallops Stuffed with Spinach and Cheese

Serves 2

PER SERVING

Calories: 324
GI: Low
Carbohydrates: 12 g.
Protein: 47 g.
Fat: 12 g.

2 ¼-pound chicken breasts,
    skinless and boneless,
    pounded thin
2 tablespoons flour
Salt and pepper to taste
¼ cup spinach soufflé (frozen)
¼ cup ricotta cheese
⅛ teaspoon nutmeg
Salt and pepper to taste
¼ cup olive oil
Juice of 1 lemon
½ cup chicken broth

This dish is wonderful for entertaining since the stuffing dresses up regular chicken and makes the dish seem more difficult to make than it actually is!

1. Sprinkle the pounded chicken breasts with flour, salt, and pepper on both sides.

2. Mix the spinach, cheese, nutmeg, and extra salt and pepper to make the filling. Spread on the chicken breasts. Roll them and secure with a toothpick.

3. Sauté the chicken in olive oil until lightly browned. Add the lemon juice and chicken broth. Cover and simmer for 15 to 20 minutes.

Making Scallops

To make chicken or veal scallops, use a rubber-headed hammer, a tool designed for pounding meat, a 5-pound weight, or the side of a heavy metal pan. Place the meat between two doubled sheets of waxed paper, pounding from the inner to outer edges. Pounding thins and tenderizes meat.

Baked Sweet Potato Sticks

These fries are good for you and make a delicious and energizing side dish that substitutes for traditional French fries. Great for kids!

1. Blanch the peeled potato slices in boiling water for 4 to 5 minutes. Dry on paper towels.

2. Sprinkle with olive oil, salt, pepper, and herbs. Bake in an aluminum pan at 350°F until crisp, about 10 minutes.

Sweet Potato Benefits

Full of fiber, potassium, and beta-carotene, sweet potatoes are an often neglected healthy and delicious vegetable—most people forget about them until Thanksgiving! Their bright orange flesh adds color to any meal, and they can be cooked like regular potatoes and taste best when baked.

---

1 large potato serves 2

PER SERVING

Calories: 104
GI: Moderate
Carbohydrates: 21 g.
Protein: 2 g.
Fat: 2 g.

---

1 large sweet potato, peeled, cut like French fries
1 tablespoon olive oil
Salt and pepper to taste
1 teaspoon thyme leaves, dried
1 teaspoon sage leaves, dried

Napa Cabbage with Asian Sauce

You can use Napa cabbage (cooked or raw) instead of pasta as a bed for sauces and meats and as a salad green. Try it steamed with various sauces. It is very low on the GI and adds fiber and antioxidants. This sauce can be adapted to your taste, from fruity to hot.

Serves 2

PER SERVING

Calories: 90
GI: Zero
Carbohydrates: 7 g.
Protein: 5 g.
Fat: 4 g.

½ Napa cabbage, cut crosswise in thin slices, separated into ribbons
¼ cup peanut oil
2 tablespoons sesame seed oil
6 scallions
1 inch gingerroot, peeled and minced
1 clove garlic, minced
½ cup soy sauce

Heat the oils and sauté the scallions, gingerroot, and garlic. Add the soy sauce and garnish. Rinse the cabbage and drain on paper towels; toss with Asian sauce.

> *Try 1 tablespoon toasted sesame seeds or the juice of half a lime as garnish.*

Pork Loin with Dried Cherries

Dried cherries, much like dried cranberries, have a uniquely sweet and tart flavor. They are a fine complement to pork, game, or poultry. The cherries plump up nicely when soaked in warm water, port wine, or any liquid. The dried cherries add a special touch to this holiday meal.

Serves 4

PER SERVING

Calories: 472
GI: Very Low
Carbohydrates: 26 g.
Protein: 55 g.
Fat: 14 g.

½ cup dried cherries
½ cup dry red wine
½ cup chicken broth
¼ cup all-purpose flour
½ teaspoon salt
½ teaspoon gingerroot, dried and ground
1 clove garlic, minced
1-½ pounds pork loin
1 tablespoon Worcestershire sauce
2 tablespoons olive oil
Salt and pepper to taste

1. Soak the cherries in the wine and chicken broth. Set aside. Spread the flour, salt, gingerroot, and garlic on a piece of waxed paper. Preheat oven to 400°F.

2. Sprinkle the Worcestershire sauce on the pork loin and roll it in the flour-spice mixture. Brown the pork in the olive oil.

3. Place the pork, cherries, and broth in a roasting pan and sprinkle with salt and pepper. Cover with aluminum foil and bake for 35 minutes.

Napa Cabbage with Eastern European Sauce

These seasonings and the sauce they produce are excellent
with stews and goulash and as a side dish.

Blanch cabbage; set aside on paper towels. Sauté the vegetables in oil or butter. Add tomatoes and spices. Place the cabbage in the sauce and simmer over low heat for 5 minutes. Garnish to taste.

> *Replace butter with olive oil to improve*
> *the healthiness of this dish.*

Hungarian Paprika

Paprika is a red spice made from ground varieties of dried peppers. The color of the paprika depends on which kind of pepper is used. You may choose to buy a more mild, delicate tasting paprika, or, if you like spicy foods, you can try a variety with more heat.

Serves 2

PER SERVING

Calories: 84
GI: Zero
Carbohydrates: 14 g.
Protein: 3 g.
Fat: 2 g.

½ Napa cabbage, cut
   crosswise in thin slices,
   separated into ribbons
1 tablespoon oil or butter
1 white onion, chopped
2 cloves garlic, chopped
1 tablespoon hot Hungarian
   paprika
Salt and pepper to taste
1-½ cups plum tomatoes,
   crushed and drained
Optional: 1 teaspoon
   caraway seeds and/or 2
   tablespoons sour cream

Pork Stuffed Wontons over Napa Cabbage

*This recipe combines Eastern and
Western flavors in a low GI, high-energy meal.*

Serves 4

PER SERVING

Calories: 635
GI: Very Low
Carbohydrates: 55 g.
Protein: 30 g.
Fat: 33 g.

2 ounces peanut oil
½ cup sweet onion, finely
    chopped
2 cloves garlic, minced
½ pound ground pork
1 ounce soy sauce
2 ounces raisins
1 ounce pine nuts, toasted
Salt and pepper to taste
24 wonton wrappers
Double recipe Napa Cabbage
    with Asian Sauce (see
    page 166)
Nonstick spray

1. Make the stuffing by sautéing onion and garlic in the peanut oil. When softened, mix in pork, stirring to break up lumps.

2. Mix in the soy sauce, raisins, pine nuts, salt, and pepper.

3. Divide the pork stuffing among wonton wrappers and moisten edges with a bit of water before folding in triangles. At this point, wontons can be stored in refrigerator for a day or frozen for a month.

4. Steam wontons in a steamer prepared with nonstick spray for 10 minutes.

5. Serve over cabbage.

Wrap It Up

Thin wonton wrappers are available at many supermarkets and all Asian markets. You can use them to make fast and easy ravioli, dumplings, or wonton soup, or you can fry the wrappers alone and top with grilled or stir-fried veggies and steak.

Shrimp and Vegetables over Napa Cabbage

*This recipe takes little time to prepare and is packed
with both flavor and energy-boosting ingredients.*

1. In a large frying pan, sauté the garlic and sesame seeds in peanut oil, stirring for 5 minutes. Add the vegetables and mix. Pour in the wine and lemon juice. Simmer to burn off alcohol; cover.

2. When the vegetables are crisp/tender, add the sherry and shrimp. Stir and cook until the shrimp turn pink. Serve with Napa Cabbage with Asian Sauce.

Serves 2

PER SERVING

Calories: 213
GI: Very Low
Carbohydrates: 15 g.
Protein: 5 g.
Fat: 11 g.

1 tablespoon peanut oil
1 clove garlic, minced
1 teaspoon sesame seeds
1 carrot, shredded
½ large zucchini, shredded
½ cup jicama, peeled and
    chopped fine
¼ cup dry white wine
1 tablespoon lemon juice
1 ounce dry sherry
½ pound raw shrimp, peeled
    and deveined
Napa Cabbage with Asian
    Sauce (see page 166)
Optional garnish: fresh
    orange sections

Veal Goulash with Napa Cabbage and Eastern European Sauce

On a cold and stormy night, make this hearty dinner.
It will warm your bones!

Serves 4

PER SERVING
(WITH RICE)

Calories: 542
GI: Low
Carbohydrates: 51 g.
Protein: 24 g.
Fat: 28 g.

1 pound veal stew meat, cut
    in large dice
Salt and pepper to taste
¼ cup vegetable oil
2 large yellow onions,
    chopped
2 cloves garlic, chopped
1 tablespoon sweet
    Hungarian paprika
1 teaspoon hot Hungarian
    paprika
2 carrots, chopped
1 stalk celery with tops,
    chopped
½ cup beer (flat)
1 cup beef broth
1 cup puréed tomatoes
¼ cup fresh parsley, chopped
1 teaspoon thyme, dried
Optional: 1 teaspoon
    caraway seeds
Optional: 1 tablespoon sour
    cream per serving
Double recipe Napa Cabbage
    with Eastern European
    Sauce (see page 167)
2 cups brown rice, cooked to
    package directions

1. Sprinkle the veal with salt and pepper. Heat oil in large stew pot and brown veal over medium heat. Stir in the onions and garlic. Sauté until soft.

2. Mix in paprikas, carrots, celery, beer, beef broth, tomatoes, and parsley. Sprinkle with thyme and caraway seeds. Cover and simmer for two hours.

3. Serve hot with Napa Cabbage and Eastern European Sauce and brown rice.

Carried Away

Caraway seeds are the dried fruit of an herb called Carum carvi and have an anise-like licorice taste. They give rye bread its distinct taste, and add flavor to pickling liquids, eastern cabbage dishes, and sauerkraut.

Veal Piquant with Ratatouille

*Using a vegetable stew as a base for meats keeps the GI of
your meal low and makes for a lovely presentation.*

1. Dress the veal with salt, pepper, and a dusting of flour. Heat the olive oil to medium-high. Sauté very quickly, about 2 minutes per side. Place on a heated serving platter.

2. Prepare the Ratatouille with White Beans. Using the pan in which the veal was cooked, add the lemon juice, capers, and herbs.

3. Stir in the chicken broth. Reduce over medium heat. Just before serving, return the veal to the pan and turn to coat with sauce. Pour the rest of the sauce over the veal and serve.

Additions and Substitutions

To add substance to this dish, you can use a mound of polenta as a base. You can also substitute chicken breasts instead of veal.

Serves 2

**PER SERVING
(NOT INCLUDING RATATOUILLE)**

Calories: 267
GI: Very Low
Carbohydrates: 5 g.
Protein: 29 g.
Fat: 14 g.

---

*Salt and pepper to taste
1 tablespoon flour
1 tablespoon olive oil
½ pound veal, sliced thin and
    pounded even thinner
Juice of ½ lemon
1 teaspoon capers
1 tablespoon fresh rosemary,
    chopped
1 tablespoon fresh parsley,
    chopped
½ cup chicken broth
Ratatouille with White Beans
    (see page 151)*

Duck Breast with Wild Mushroom Sauce over Wild Rice or Polenta

If you know a mycologist or visit some farmers' markets,
you can get wonderful wild mushrooms.
Otherwise use shitakes or brown mushrooms available in the supermarket.

Serves 2

PER SERVING

Calories: 578
GI: Low
Carbohydrates: 34 g.
Protein: 48 g.
Fat: 23 g.

2 duck breasts, boneless,
    skinless
2 tablespoons flour
Salt and pepper to taste
½ teaspoon thyme
⅛ teaspoon cayenne pepper
½ teaspoon Chinese 5-spice
    powder
2 tablespoons canola oil
1 cup wild rice, prepared to
    package directions
1 tablespoon butter
4 shallots
1 cup wild or exotic
    mushrooms, cleaned and
    coarsely chopped
½ cup chicken broth
2 tablespoons Apple Jack or
    Calvados (Spanish apple
    brandy)
1 tablespoon fresh rosemary,
    or 1 teaspoon dried

1. Coat the duck breasts in a mixture of flour, salt, pepper, thyme, cayenne, and 5-spice powder. Heat the canola oil to medium-high and sauté the duck for 4 to 5 minutes per side to brown.

2. Remove the duck to a warm serving platter. Cook the wild rice.

3. Using the same pan, stir in the butter and shallots. Sauté for 3 to 4 minutes. Add the mushrooms and toss to coat with butter.

4. Stir in the chicken broth, Apple Jack or Calvados, and rosemary. Return the duck to the pan. Cover and cook for 5 minutes.

> ♥ *You can substitute olive oil for butter in this recipe.* ♥

Chicken Breast with Snap Peas and White Beans

The snap peas and white beans add to the protein in this recipe and provide a shot of energy that will last for hours. Aside from being a convenient one-pot meal, this is a delectable dish!

1. Cut the chicken in large chunks; sprinkle with salt and pepper. Sauté the chicken and garlic in the olive oil over medium heat.

2. Add scallions and toss with the snap peas; cook for 4 minutes.

3. Stir in the rest of the ingredients; cover and simmer for 10 minutes and serve.

Serves 2

PER SERVING

Calories: 571
GI: Very Low
Carbohydrates: 44 g.
Protein: 54 g.
Fat: 23 g.

½ pound chicken breasts, boneless and skinless
Salt and pepper to taste
1 ounce olive oil
2 cloves garlic, chopped
10 fresh scallions, chopped
1 cup snap peas, chopped
1 tablespoon fresh rosemary, or 1 teaspoon dried
4 fresh basil leaves, or 1 teaspoon dried
2 tablespoons dry white vermouth
1 cup canned whole tomatoes, drained
13-ounce can white beans, drained
1 teaspoon red pepper flakes, or to taste

Scrod Filets with Crispy Potatoes

*Scrod is wonderful in this dish with potatoes, makes a fine addition
to fish soup, and can be baked, broiled, sautéed, or fried.*

Serves 2

Per Serving

Calories: 500
GI: Moderate
Carbohydrates: 34 g.
Protein: 25 g.
Fat: 31 g.

*1 large Idaho or Yukon gold
    potato, peeled and sliced
    thin
½ Bermuda or Vidalia onion,
    sliced thin
2 ounces olive oil
Salt and pepper to taste
¼ teaspoon paprika
1 teaspoon thyme,
    dried, crumbled, or 1
    tablespoon fresh
8 ounces scrod filet
Juice of ½ lemon
1 teaspoon butter
Nonstick spray*

1. Toss the potato and onion in a mixture of olive oil, salt, pepper, paprika, and thyme. Preheat oven to 375°F.

2. Prepare an 8" pie plate with nonstick spray. Spread the potatoes and onions in the plate and bake for 35 to 40 minutes, or until the top is crisply brown and the inside layer of potatoes is soft.

3. Place the fish on top, sprinkle with lemon juice, and dot with butter. Bake for another 10 minutes, or until the fish flakes.

 You can dot the fish in this recipe with heart-healthy margarine instead of butter to lower the fat content.

Scrod Basics

Scrod is the name for a young codfish, although some say it can also be used to describe young haddock or similar tasting fish. It is mild, tender, and very versatile, and it is a favorite in England and New England for fish and chips.

Corn-Crusted Salmon with Parsley and Radish Topping

This is a festive way to prepare salmon and very pretty with the colorful green parsley and red radishes.

1. Mix the radishes, parsley, olive oil, vinegar, and celery salt. Set aside.

2. Make sure the salmon has no pin bones; sprinkle with lemon juice. Mix together the cornmeal, milk, dill, olive oil, and red pepper flakes. Spread on the salmon and rest it in the refrigerator for ½ hour.

3. Set oven at 350°F. Prepare a baking dish or metal sheet with nonstick spray. Place salmon on the baking dish or sheet.

4. Bake the salmon for 20 minutes, or until the topping is brown and the salmon flakes. Serve with radish-parsley topping.

> *Substitute nonfat milk for 2% milk in the topping for the salmon in this recipe.*

Serves 2

PER SERVING

Calories: 371
GI: Very Low
Carbohydrates: 10 g.
Protein: 36 g.
Fat: 21 g.

4 radishes, thinly sliced
½ cup parsley, Italian flat-leaf, minced
1 tablespoon olive oil
2 tablespoons red wine vinegar
½ teaspoon celery salt
2 salmon filets, about 6 ounces each
1 tablespoon lemon juice
¼ cup cornmeal
¼ cup 2% milk
½ teaspoon dill, dried
3 tablespoons olive oil
Red pepper flakes to taste
Nonstick spray

chapter 12

Diet-Friendly Meals

Filet Mignon and Roasted Red Pepper Wraps

When you are cutting calories and carbohydrates,
yet you want loads of flavor, this is a great way to do it!
You will get carbohydrates from the pepper and lettuce.

1. Lay the lettuce out on paper towels. Skim the olive oil in the bottom of a medium frying pan; set on medium heat. Sauté the onion and garlic for 1 to 2 minutes.

2. Sprinkle salt and pepper on the filet mignon and sauté quickly.

3. Place a piece of cheese on each lettuce leaf; pile on onions, garlic, and filet mignon. Sprinkle with Worcestershire sauce and Tabasco sauce. Add roasted red peppers. Wrap and serve.

> ♥   *Omit the cheese in this recipe to cut back on calories.*   ♥

Serves 2

PER SERVING

Calories: 415
GI: Zero
Carbohydrates: 7 g.
Protein: 44 g.
Fat: 31 g.

---

4 large, outside leaves of romaine lettuce
1 tablespoon olive oil
1 sweet onion, such as Vidalia, chopped fine
1 clove garlic, minced
Salt and pepper to taste
8-ounce filet mignon, sliced thinly
2 ounces roasted red pepper, chopped (from a jar is fine)
1 teaspoon Worcestershire sauce
½ teaspoon Tabasco sauce, or to taste
4 slices white American cheese

London Broil with Grilled Vegetables

London broil is a lot cheaper than filet mignon and is still very tasty.
You can use meat tenderizer on it or marinate to add to the flavor.
This meal is perfect when done on the grill with the veggies on skewers.

1. In a small bowl, mix the olive oil, vinegar, steak sauce, and seasonings and set aside. Skewer the vegetables.

2. Brush the vegetables with the dressing. Toss the London broil in the rest of the dressing to coat and skewer.

3. Heat grill to 350°F and roast the vegetables and meat to the desired level of doneness.

Keep Your Eye on the Beef

Beef is high-quality protein, but beware—when you eat too much of it or have it with rich sauces, the caloric count skyrockets.

Serves 2

PER SERVING

Calories: 354
GI: Very Low
Carbohydrates: 26 g.
Protein: 39 g.
Fat: 12 g.

---

2 tablespoons olive oil
1 teaspoon red wine vinegar
1 tablespoon steak sauce
1 teaspoon salt, or to taste
1 teaspoon red pepper flakes, or to taste
1 zucchini, cut in 1-inch chunks
1 orange or yellow pepper, seeded and cored, cut in quarters
2 sweet onions, cut in thick chunks
4 cherry tomatoes
½ pound London broil, cut in chunks
4 wooden skewers, presoaked for 30 minutes

Roast Leg of Veal

Serves 8

PER SERVING

Calories: 174
GI: Zero
Carbohydrates: 1 g.
Protein: 22 g.
Fat: 7 g.

5-pound veal leg roast, shank half of the leg, bone in
1 tablespoon prepared mustard, Dijon style
2 tablespoons all-purpose flour
1 tablespoon butter, at room temperature
1 teaspoon dried sage, crumbled
2 teaspoons dried rosemary, crumbled
Salt and freshly ground black pepper to taste
1 cup chicken broth
½ cup dry white wine

It may take a trip on the Internet to find a veal roast; however, if you can get a young one, it's fabulous. A crisp salad, asparagus, or broccoli make excellent accompaniments.

1. Make sure the veal is well trimmed and has no skin on it. Set oven at 400°F. Make a paste of the mustard, flour, butter, herbs, salt, and pepper. Coat the veal with the mustard mixture.

2. Place veal in a roasting pan and place in the hot, preheated oven. Roast for 15 minutes. Turn down heat and baste with ¼ cup chicken broth and in 15 minutes with ¼ cup wine.

3. Reduce heat to 325°F. Continue to roast and baste the meat for another 45 minutes, or until the internal temperature reaches 150°F.

4. Let the meat rest on a platter for 15 minutes before carving. Serve with pan juices; if dry, add ½ cup boiling water to pan and whisk.

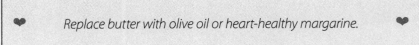

Replace butter with olive oil or heart-healthy margarine.

Veal Stew with Peppers

Veal is wonderful with any vegetable and is great when flavored with lemon, garlic, and almost all herbs. This dish is delicious over spaghetti, polenta, or rice or served as a hero sandwich.

1. Sprinkle the veal with salt, pepper, and flour. Heat the olive oil in a stew pot. Quickly sear the veal; remove and set it aside.

2. Sauté the onion and garlic in the remaining oil. If dry, add 1 tablespoon more oil. Stir in the herbs, tomato sauce, and wine.

3. Return the veal to the pot; cover and simmer over low heat for 45 minutes. Add mushrooms at the end of cooking time. Check for tenderness before serving. If necessary, simmer for another 10 minutes.

What Is Veal?

Veal is young beef that is the meat of the male offspring of dairy cows. It is naturally white when cooked and as a raw meat should be pale pink, not red. The difference in color is because younger cows have less iron in their muscles than older beef cows.

Serves 4

Per Serving

Calories: 309
GI: Zero
Carbohydrates: 7 g.
Protein: 29 g.
Fat: 17 g.

---

1 pound veal stew meat, boneless
Salt and pepper to taste
1 tablespoon flour
1 tablespoon olive oil
½ cup yellow onion, chopped
2 cloves garlic, minced
2 teaspoons sage leaves, dried
1 teaspoon oregano, dried
1 cup tomato sauce
¼ cup dry red wine
Optional: 1 cup mushrooms, sliced

Poached Mediterranean Chicken with Olives, Tomatoes, and Herbs

Poaching a skinless, boneless chicken breast is a calorie-conscious and practical mode of cooking. The chicken does not dry out as it does when grilled or broiled, and no oil is necessary. You don't get a lovely brown color, but it's delicious anyway.

Serves 2

PER SERVING

Calories: 330
GI: Zero
Carbohydrates: 11 g.
Protein: 43 g.
Fat: 12 g.

1 cup low-salt chicken broth
1 large fresh tomato, cored and chopped
4 ounces pearl onions, fresh or frozen
4 to 6 cloves roasted garlic (see page 247)
10 spicy black olives, such as Kalamata or Sicilian
10 green olives, pitted (no pimientos)
½ teaspoon oregano leaves, dried, crumbled
1 teaspoon mint leaves, dried, crumbled
4 fresh basil leaves, torn
2 4-ounce chicken breasts, boneless and skinless
Salt and pepper to taste
½ teaspoon lemon zest
4 sprigs parsley

1. Make the poaching liquid by placing all of the ingredients except for the chicken, salt and pepper, lemon zest, and parsley in a large saucepan. Bring to a boil; reduce heat and simmer for 5 minutes.

2. Add the chicken, salt and pepper. Simmer for another 8 minutes and add lemon zest. Sprinkle with parsley and serve.

Choosing Tomatoes

In season, use vine ripe tomotoes. Off-season, use quality canned rather than greenhouse tomatoes. Tomatoes should be aromatic; tomatoes with no aroma will have no taste. Avoid tomatoes with leathery, dark patches—this is a sign of blossom-end rot.

Filet Mignon

When you need a protein fix, mix in some carbohydrates,
like the mushrooms in this recipe, to boost your energy and brainpower.

1. Sprinkle the filet mignon with salt and pepper. Heat a heavy fry pan prepared with nonstick spray over medium-high flame.

2. Sear the filet mignon quickly on both sides. Stir in the mushrooms. Remove beef when at desired level of doneness. Add the liquids and bring to a boil. Pour the sauce over the beef. Serve hot with optional aioli.

Serves 2

PER SERVING

Calories: 266
GI: Zero
Carbohydrates: 3 g.
Protein: 33 g.
Fat: 11 g.

8-ounce filet mignon
Salt and pepper to taste
Nonstick spray
½ cup white button
*   mushrooms, chopped*
2 ounces dry red wine
2 ounces beef broth
Optional: 2 teaspoons aioli
*   (see page 238)*

Poached Chicken with Pears and Herbs

Any seasonal fresh fruit will make a dish very special. If you have some fruit brandy or eau-de-vie, a splash will also add to the flavor. Pears go very well with all poultry. Try this for a quick treat and double the recipe for company.

Prepare the poaching liquid by mixing the first 5 ingredients and bringing to a boil in a saucepan. Salt and pepper the chicken and add to the pan. Simmer slowly for 10 minutes. Serve with pears on top of each piece.

Serves 2

PER SERVING

Calories: 307
GI: Very Low
Carbohydrates: 15 g.
Protein: 41 g.
Fat: 9 g.

1 ripe pear, peeled, cored, and
*   cut in chunks*
2 shallots, minced
½ cup dry white wine
1 teaspoon rosemary, dried,
*   or 1 tablespoon fresh*
1 teaspoon thyme, dried, or
*   1 tablespoon fresh*
2 ½-pound chicken breasts,
*   boneless and skinless*
Salt and pepper to taste

Grilled San Francisco-Style Chicken

*This is a quick chef's delight. It's excellent, and everyone
at your table will ask "what is in this?"*

Serves 4

PER SERVING

Calories: 95
GI: Zero
Carbohydrates: 7 g.
Protein: 40 g.
Fat: 10 g.

1 tablespoon olive oil
1 tablespoon Dijon-style
    mustard
2 tablespoons raspberry
    white wine vinegar
Celery salt and pepper to
    taste
1 small chicken, about 2-½ to
    3 pounds, cut in quarters

1. Heat grill to 400°F. In a small bowl, mix the olive oil, mustard, and vinegar. Sprinkle the chicken with celery salt and pepper.

2. Paint the skin side of the chicken with the mustard mixture. Spray a few drops of olive oil on the bone side.

3. Grill the chicken, bone side to flame, for 15 minutes. Reduce heat to 325°F; cover and cook for 15 minutes.

Braised Chicken with Citrus

*Chicken is wonderfully flavored by lemons, oranges, and grapefruits.
Try it, and use the sauce over rice!*

Serves 2

PER SERVING

Calories: 274
GI: Very Low
Carbohydrates: 7 g.
Protein: 40 g.
Fat: 10 g.

¼ cup orange juice
¼ cup grapefruit juice, fresh
    or unsweetened
1 tablespoon orange
    Curacao, or other liqueur
1 teaspoon savory herb, dried
½ teaspoon lemon zest
1 teaspoon extra-virgin olive
    oil
Salt and pepper to taste
½ pound chicken breasts,
    boneless and skinless, cut
    in chunks

Make poaching liquid with the first 6 ingredients. Sprinkle the chicken with salt and pepper. Poach for 10 minutes and serve over rice or chilled in a salad.

Stewed Chicken with Garlic

This is an old-fashioned French country meal. You can opt to soak up the juices with toasted French bread, serve it over rice, or just eat it plain.

Serves 4

Per Serving

Calories: 142
GI: Zero
Carbohydrates: 4 g.
Protein: 9 g.
Fat: 8 g.

1. Melt the butter in a large pan over medium heat. Rinse the chicken, pat it dry, and cut into quarters. Sprinkle with salt and pepper. Sauté until lightly brown.

2. Add the onions, garlic, celery, wine, thyme, and chicken broth. Reduce heat to a simmer and cover. Cook for 35 minutes, or until very tender and fragrant.

3. Place the chicken on a platter. Whisk in the flour and pour sauce over the chicken.

1 tablespoon butter
1 whole chicken
Salt and pepper to taste
16 pearl onions
1 head of garlic, roasted,
   cloves separated, garlic
   squeezed out
2 stalks celery, chopped
½ cup dry white wine
1 teaspoon thyme
½ cup chicken broth
1 tablespoon Wondra
   quick-blending flour (for
   thickening the stew)
Optional: Serve with
   potatoes, rice, or noodles

> ❤ *Substitute olive oil for butter to lighten*
> *the fat content in this French recipe.* ❤

Grilled Tuna Steak with Vegetables and Pine Nuts

*Grilled tuna is a favorite of dieters. The Asian vegetables
in this recipe add some carbohydrates necessary for good health.*

Serves 2

PER SERVING

Calories: 277
GI: Zero
Carbohydrates: 25 g.
Protein: 18 g.
Fat: 13 g.

1 cup Napa cabbage, shredded
½ cup pea pods, chopped
*   coarsely*
½ cup carrots, shredded
¼ cup pine nuts, toasted
3 tablespoons tomato sauce
2 tuna steaks, ¼ pound each
1 teaspoon sesame oil
1 teaspoon lime juice
Salt and pepper to taste

1. Poach the vegetables in the tomato sauce for 8 minutes or until crisp-tender. Add the pine nuts and set aside.

2. Set grill on medium-high. Spread the tuna with sesame oil, lime juice, salt, and pepper. Grill for 4 minutes per side for medium.

3. Serve with tomato-poached vegetables.

Grilled Rib Lamb Chops with Garlic and Citrus

Young lamb is a great party dish and is perfect when cooked medium rare.

Serves 2

PER SERVING

Calories: 513
GI: Zero
Carbohydrates: 0 g.
Protein: 68 g.
Fat: 24 g.

2 teaspoons olive oil
½ lemon, juice and zest
1 tablespoon grapefruit juice
1 to 2 cloves garlic, minced
1 teaspoon dried rosemary, or
*   1 tablespoon fresh*
Salt and pepper to taste
8 baby rib lamb chops, about
*   ½ inch each, well trimmed*
2 tablespoons white
*   vermouth, for basting*

1. Using a mortar and pestle, mash the olive oil, lemon juice and zest, grapefruit juice, garlic, rosemary, salt, and pepper.

2. Make sure all fat is removed from the lamb chops. Coat lamb chops with the garlic mixture and let rest in the refrigerator for 1 hour.

3. Heat grill to high. Place chops over high flame until seared on one side. Baste with vermouth and turn after 3 minutes. Baste again and reduce heat. Cover the grill and let chops roast for 8 minutes.

Salmon Steaks with Asparagus in Light Egg Sauce

You can keep your glycemic index low by consuming large amounts of high-quality carbohydrates, like the vegetables in this dish. The soy sauce in this meal adds a great deal of rich, smoky, and nutty flavor.

Serves 2

PER SERVING

Calories: 224
GI: Very Low
Carbohydrates: 7 g.
Protein: 30 g.
Fat: 15 g.

*2 fresh salmon steaks,
    ½ pound each*
*½ pound fresh or frozen
    asparagus, steamed*
1 tablespoon soy sauce
*2 tablespoons low-fat
    mayonnaise*
½ lemon, juice and zest
½ teaspoon garlic powder
*½ teaspoon red hot pepper
    sauce, or to taste*
*1 egg, hard-boiled and
    chopped*

1. Broil or grill the salmon steaks, 4 minutes per side. Plate, surrounding with asparagus.

2. Mix the soy sauce, mayonnaise, lemon juice and zest, garlic powder, hot pepper sauce, and chopped egg together to make a sauce. Drizzle over salmon and asparagus.

Testing Egg Freshness

To test whether or not an egg is fresh, immerse it in a pan of cool, salted water. If it sinks to the bottom, it is fresh. If it rises to the surface, it is spoiled. If the eggs in your refrigerator are approaching or have passed their freshness date, always perform this test before using the eggs.

Salmon and Broccoli Stir-Fry

This is a quick and easy supper, in addition to being good for you.
You can blanch the broccoli in advance.

Serves 2

PER SERVING

Calories: 273
GI: Zero
Carbohydrates: 7 g.
Protein: 25 g.
Fat: 6 g.

½ pound broccoli florets
½ pound salmon filet, skin
* removed*
1 tablespoon canola oil
1 teaspoon Asian sesame oil
1 teaspoon gingerroot,
* minced*
2 slices pickled ginger,
* chopped*
1 clove garlic, minced
1 teaspoon hoisin sauce
Garnish of 5 scallions,
* chopped*
Optional: 1 cup brown rice

1. Blanch the broccoli in boiling water for 5 minutes; drain.

2. Toss the broccoli and salmon over medium-high heat with the canola oil and sesame oil. Cook, stirring for 3 to 4 minutes.

3. Add the gingerroot, pickled ginger, garlic, and hoisin sauce and serve over rice, garnished with scallions.

Food Safety

When preparing a dish that lists fish, seafood, or poultry as one of the ingredients, be sure to keep the fish, seafood, or chicken ice cold during preparation to ensure food safety. If you will be doing a lot of handling or if the food will be on the counter for a long time, keep a bowl with ice nearby to place the ingredients in while you are tending to other steps of the recipe.

Roast Stuffed Striped Bass

This is very festive and can serve a mob by multiplying the recipe.

1. Place everything but the striped bass in the food processor or blender. Pulse until well crumbled.

2. Set oven on 350°F. Place striped bass on a baking sheet. Spread stuffing on fish.

3. Bake the fish for 12 to 15 minutes, or until the stuffing is well browned.

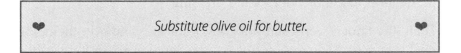

Substitute olive oil for butter.

Stripers

Striped bass are native to a large portion of the East Coast and range as far south as northern Florida. The fish has lean, white meat and a mild flavor and is especially tasty when stuffed with vegetables and bread crumbs or grilled.

Serves 2

PER SERVING

Calories: 395
GI: Low
Carbohydrates: 22 g.
Protein: 36 g.
Fat: 19 g.

2 slices whole grain bread, toasted
1 stalk celery, chopped finely
¼ cup parsley, chopped
2 tablespoons unsalted butter, melted
½ cup canned water chestnuts
1 tablespoon lemon juice
Salt and pepper to taste
¾ pound filet of striped bass, skin on

Fresh Tuna Salad a la Niçoise

*Fresh tuna makes a classic Italian antipasto or salad.
This great salad is made with baby green beans
(haricots verts) and small new potatoes.*

Serves 2

PER SERVING

Calories: 443
GI: Zero
Carbohydrates: 61 g.
Protein: 32 g.
Fat: 7 g.

*1 teaspoon olive oil
½ pound fresh tuna steak
Salt and pepper to taste
4 small new potatoes
½ pound haricot verts
Juice of ½ lemon
1 ounce red wine vinegar
1 teaspoon Worcestershire
     sauce
½ teaspoon Dijon-style mustard
¼ cup extra-virgin olive oil*

1. Brush the tuna steaks with olive oil and sprinkle with salt and pepper. Sauté quickly over medium-high heat for 3 minutes per side and set the tuna aside.

2. In a saucepan, bring 2 cups water to a boil and cook the potatoes and haricot verts together. Cut cooked potatoes in halves. Mix the rest of the ingredients in the blender for the dressing.

3. Drain the haricot verts and potatoes; pour dressing over them, tossing gently to coat. Slice and add the tuna. Serve at room temperature or chill.

Pasta Salad with Vegetables

*When you mix pasta made with slow-digesting semolina with
low GI carbohydrates such as fibrous vegetables, the GI goes even lower.
This is a light lunch or supper for when you plan to be physically active.*

Serves 2

PER SERVING

Calories: 624
GI: Low
Carbohydrates: 99 g.
Protein: 17 g.
Fat: 20 g.

*1 cup cooked pasta, such as
     small shells or orecchiette
1 cup fresh green beans,
     blanched
6 scallions, chopped
½ sweet red pepper, cored,
     seeded, and chopped
4 ounces French dressing (see
     page 92)
½ cup fresh Italian parsley,
     chopped*

Mix all ingredients in a serving bowl; chill and serve.

Baked Filet of Sole with Shrimp Sauce and Artichokes

The varieties of sole are daunting. There's gray, lemon, Dover, and more. When you are buying sole, make sure that it smells like fresh milk. Get whatever is cheapest—it will taste pretty much the same from lemon to gray to Dover. All taste delicious when fresh!

Serves 2

PER SERVING

Calories: 368
GI: Very Low
Carbohydrates: 20 g.
Protein: 43 g.
Fat: 13 g.

5 medium shrimp, cooked
1 shallot, chopped
¼ cup low-fat mayonnaise
¼ teaspoon dill, dried
2 tablespoons orange juice
1 9-ounce package frozen artichoke hearts
2 6-ounce sole filets
Salt and pepper to taste
4 tablespoons fine dry bread crumbs
Nonstick spray

1. Preheat oven to 375°F. Pulse the shrimp, shallot, mayonnaise, dill, and orange juice in the blender. Set the sauce aside.

2. Cook the frozen artichokes to package directions. Place sole on a baking sheet prepared with nonstick spray. Sprinkle the filets with salt and pepper. Arrange the artichokes around the sole. Spoon sauce over all. Sprinkle with bread crumbs.

3. Bake for 15 minutes, or until the sole is hot and bubbling and the artichokes crisply browned on top.

Artichokes

Artichokes are the flowers of a large plant and are available November through May. There are two varieties—those with thorns ("unarmed") those known as "Roman," and the prickly type, which have little thorns at the triangular tip of each leaf. The soft heart or center of the artichoke can be eaten raw or cooked sprinkled with olive oil, salt, and pepper.

Lettuce-Wrapped Turkey with Cranberry Mayonnaise and Apples

Using lettuce for a wrap is an excellent way to lower your GI.
This is a terrific way to use up Thanksgiving leftovers in a healthy way.

Serves 1

PER SERVING

Calories: 325
GI: Very Low
Carbohydrates: 17 g.
Protein: 32 g.
Fat: 15 g.

2 large romaine lettuce leaves
2 teaspoons low-fat
    mayonnaise
1 teaspoon cranberry sauce,
    jelled
1 teaspoon prepared
    horseradish
¼ pound deli or leftover
    turkey, diced
½ stalk celery, chopped fine
1 slice onion, chopped fine
½ tart apple, cored and
    chopped fine
1 tablespoon walnuts,
    toasted and chopped

1. Lay the lettuce leaves on a work surface. In a small bowl, mix together the mayonnaise, cranberry sauce, and horseradish.

2. Place the sliced turkey on top of the lettuce leaves. Mix the celery, onion, apple, and walnuts with the cranberry mayonnaise. Spread on the turkey and roll up the wrap.

Wild about Walnuts

Walnuts are one of the best things you can consume for your body. Like salmon and other cold-water fish, walnuts contain omega-3 fatty acids, which lower cholesterol and blood pressure and supply fat that can even help your brain function!

Baked Ricotta Cheese Casserole with Hot Peppers and Vegetables

This is a very tasty way to get your children to consume the calcium they need.

1. Heat the olive oil in a nonstick pan. Sauté the vegetables in olive oil for 5 minutes. Preheat the oven to 350ºF.

2. Mix the beaten eggs with the cheeses, herbs, salt, and pepper. Stir in the vegetables. Prepare a gratin pan with nonstick spray. Add the cheese and vegetables mixture. Spread top with tomato sauce and bake for 30 minutes. Serve hot, topped with your garnish of choice.

Cutting Down on Salt

Ricotta cheese has a naturally high salt content so you may want to keep that in mind when adding additional salt for flavoring.

Serves 4

PER SERVING

Calories: 125
GI: Very Low
Carbohydrates: 4 g.
Protein: 5 g.
Fat: 11 g.

---

1 tablespoon olive oil
½ cup sweet red onion, chopped
1 medium zucchini, chopped
1 medium carrot, peeled and grated
2 Jalapeño peppers, seeded and minced
2 beaten eggs
1 pound ricotta cheese
1 teaspoon dried oregano
½ cup fresh basil
Salt and pepper to taste
2 tablespoons Parmesan cheese, grated
1 cup tomato sauce
Optional garnishes: 1 tablespoon capers or green peppercorns
Nonstick spray

Mini Spinach Casserole with Ricotta Cheese, Brown Rice, and Ham

This is a delicious way to keep your GI low while getting nutrients.

Purée the spinach and ricotta in the blender. Preheat oven to 300°F. Mix all ingredients together in a 9" pie pan and bake for 20 minutes.

Serves 2

PER SERVING

Calories: 342
GI: Low
Carbohydrates: 32 g.
Protein: 16 g.
Fat: 19 g.

2 cups fresh baby spinach
½ cup low-fat ricotta cheese
Salt and pepper to taste
1 cup brown rice, cooked
¼ cup Italian dressing (see page 92)
1 ounce Virginia Ham, chopped

Pork Tenderloin with Caraway Sauerkraut

Caraway is a popular flavor in Scandinavian and Eastern European cooking. It is excellent with veal and pork. Tenderloin of pork is lean, moist, and delicious. It is very low in calories and a real treat with the sauerkraut.

1. Heat the oil in a frying pan over medium heat. Sprinkle the pork tenderloin with salt, pepper, and flour. Sauté the pork over medium heat for 4 minutes; turn the pork and add onions.

2. Continue to sauté until the pork is lightly browned on both sides and the onions have softened slightly.

3. Add the chicken broth, sauerkraut, and caraway seeds. Cover and simmer for 25 minutes. Pork should be pink.

Serves 2

PER SERVING

Calories: 309
GI: Zero
Carbohydrates: 4 g.
Protein: 36 g.
Fat: 15 g.

1 teaspoon olive oil
Salt and pepper to taste
1 teaspoon Wondra flour
8 ounces pork tenderloin
2 medium red onions, chopped
¼ cup low-salt chicken broth
8 ounces sauerkraut, drained
1 teaspoon caraway seeds

Chapter 13
Balanced Family Dinners

Turkey Meat Loaf with Thanksgiving Herbs

*Meat loaf is a creative way to include vegetables
in your children's meals. Even grown-ups who refuse to eat
vegetables will eat them and love them in this recipe.*

1. Using a large frying pan, sauté the onion, garlic, carrot, zucchini, and celery in the olive oil. Start soaking the corn bread stuffing in the chicken broth.

2. Beat the eggs and mix with the tomato paste, Worcestershire sauce, cloves, salt, pepper, and herbs. Add to the vegetable mixture. Remove from heat. Cool slightly and stir in the soaked corn bread stuffing. (If the stuffing is seasoned, do not add salt.)

3. Stir the turkey into the egg-vegetable-stuffing mixture and mix well. Pour into a loaf pan that you have prepared with nonstick spray. Bake at 350°F for 1 hour. Serve with cranberry sauce or relish.

Serves 4

PER SERVING

Calories: 378
GI: Very Low
Carbohydrates: 17 g.
Protein: 28 g.
Fat: 22 g.

2 tablespoons olive oil
1 yellow onion, minced
1 clove garlic, minced
1 large carrot, peeled and
    grated
1 zucchini, grated
1 stalk celery, chopped finely
1 cup corn bread stuffing
1 cup chicken broth
1 teaspoon tomato paste
1 teaspoon Worcestershire
    sauce
¼ teaspoon cloves, ground
1 teaspoon thyme, dried
Salt and pepper to taste
1 teaspoon sage leaves, dried
2 eggs, beaten
1 pound ground turkey
Nonstick spray

Turkey Roll with Spinach and Cheese

You can use turkey in so many ways that your family will love.
A grilled turkey leg and thigh is delicious on a summer night,
as is this turkey roll. The finished design of a circle within
a circle makes an attractive presentation.

1. Place the turkey breast between several sheets of waxed paper. Using a rubber hammer or meat mallet, flatten the turkey breast until it's about ½ inch thick. Sprinkle with salt and pepper.

2. Preheat the oven to 325°F. Spread the spinach on the turkey. Sprinkle with lemon juice, dot with shredded American cheese, and sprinkle with olive oil. Roll and skewer with metal poultry pins.

3. Sprinkle with Parmesan cheese. Wrap the top with bacon and roast until the internal temperature reaches 150°F. Let rest before carving.

> *Substitute vegetarian bacon for regular bacon*
> *here and replace regular American cheese with*
> *low-fat American cheese.*

Serves 4

Per Serving

Calories: 432
GI: Zero
Carbohydrates: 6 g.
Protein: 60 g.
Fat: 18 g.

1-½ pounds turkey breast,
    boneless and skinless
Salt and pepper to taste
1 10-ounce package spinach
    soufflé, thawed
1 tablespoon lemon juice
2 slices white American
    cheese, shredded
1 teaspoon olive oil
2 tablespoons Parmesan
    cheese, grated
2 slices bacon

Roast Turkey Breast

When you roast a turkey breast, you can serve a crowd or just the family and then have lots of extra meat for salads, lunch, or dinner the next day.

PER SERVING

Calories: 509
GI: Zero
(without stuffing),
Low (with stuffing)
Carbohydrates: 20 g.
Protein: 59 g.
Fat: 20 g.

1 tablespoon butter or heart-
   healthy margarine
1 medium yellow onion,
   chopped
1 stalk celery, chopped
½ cup fresh parsley, Italian
   flat-leaf variety
3 tart apples, peeled, cored,
   and chopped
1 cup walnuts, toasted and
   chopped
1 medium orange, skin and
   seeds removed, cut in
   small pieces
1 cup corn bread crumbs
   (your own or commercial
   corn bread stuffing)
1 tablespoon rosemary, dried,
   or 2 tablespoons fresh
4-pound turkey breast, skin
   on, bone in
Salt and pepper to taste
1 teaspoon olive oil
1 cup cranberry juice

1. Make the stuffing by melting the butter and sautéing the onion, celery, parsley, and apples for 5 minutes, or until soft. Mix in the walnuts and ½ of the orange pieces. Continue to mix and add the bread crumbs and rosemary. If very dry, add a bit of water.

2. Place the stuffing on a large piece of aluminum foil and reserve. Preheat the oven to 350°F. Push the rest of the orange between the turkey skin and flesh. Sprinkle the turkey skin with salt and pepper. Rub with olive oil.

3. Place the turkey breast over the stuffing and make a boat with the foil. Roast the turkey for 2-½ hours, basting every 20 minutes with cranberry juice. Let rest for 10 minutes before serving.

The Multitalented Turkey

Turkey is a healthy, lean meat that is packed with protein and contains vitamin B6, which helps your body produce energy. These days it is easy to incorporate turkey into your diet because you can buy turkey cutlets, ground turkey, and turkey breasts instead of just a whole turkey.

Fried Chicken with Cornmeal Crust

Coarsely grated cornmeal makes an excellent crust for fried chicken. There are people who use corn muffin mix as the coating for their chicken. While that's fine, it's more wholesome to make your own crust.

1. Soak the chicken in buttermilk for 15 minutes. On a piece of waxed paper, mix the cornmeal, baking powder, salt, and pepper. Coat the chicken with the cornmeal mixture.

2. In a large frying pan, heat the oil to 350°F. Fry for 8 to 10 minutes per side. Drain on paper towels.

Serves 4

PER SERVING

Calories: 265
GI: Low
Carbohydrates: 9 g.
Protein: 42 g.
Fat: 9 g.

4 half-breasts chicken, 4 ounces each, boneless and skinless
½ cup buttermilk
½ cup coarse cornmeal
1 teaspoon baking powder
½ teaspoon salt
Freshly ground pepper to taste
½ inch canola or other oil in a deep pan for frying

Turkey Meatballs

These baked meatballs turn out delicious and are far less fattening than fried meatballs. Serve with a flavorful sauce such as a tomato artichoke sauce.

1. Mix all but the bread crumbs in the food processor or blender, adding ingredients one by one.

2. Form into balls and roll in bread crumbs. Bake for 35 minutes at 325°F; turn once.

3. Serve with a tomato-based sauce.

Serves 4 (16 meatballs)

PER SERVING

Calories: 476
GI: Very Low
Carbohydrates: 45 g.
Protein: 35 g.
Fat: 20 g.

2 slices whole grain bread
½ cup 2% milk
2 eggs
½ cup chili sauce
½ cup yellow onion, chopped
2 cloves garlic, minced
1 teaspoon oregano, dried
½ teaspoon red pepper flakes
¼ cup Parmesan cheese, finely grated
1 pound ground turkey meat
1 cup fine, dry bread crumbs

> ❤ *Substitute nonfat milk for 2% milk.* ❤

Scalloped Potato and Sausage Casserole with Greens

This recipe is another creative way to get your family to eat vegetables. Among the bits of sausage, your family will hardly notice them. The spices in the sausage will perfume the potatoes and veggies.

Serves 4

PER SERVING

Calories: 277
GI: Moderate
Carbohydrates: 50 g.
Protein: 13 g.
Fat: 5 g.

1 teaspoon vegetable oil
8 ounces lean pork breakfast
    sausage, crumbled
1 yellow onion, sliced
1 small zucchini, ends
    removed, diced
10-ounce package chopped
    frozen spinach, thawed
    and squeezed of moisture
¼ teaspoon nutmeg
Salt and pepper to taste
2 Idaho or other russet
    potatoes, peeled and
    sliced thinly
¼ cup Parmesan cheese,
    grated
⅔ cup 2% milk
½ cup bread crumbs
Nonstick spray

1. Heat the oil in a large frying pan and sauté the sausage, onion, and zucchini. Stir to break up the sausage and mix well.

2. Stir in the spinach, nutmeg, salt, and pepper. Set aside.

3. Prepare a 9" pie plate with nonstick spray. Cover the bottom with sliced potatoes, add the sausage filling, and cover the top with the rest of the potatoes. Sprinkle with cheese and add milk.

4. Cover the top with bread crumbs; press down to moisten with milk. Bake for 50 minutes at 325°F, or until the potatoes are soft.

> *Substitute nonfat milk for 2% milk and replace sausage with vegetarian sausage.*

Stewed Chicken with Vegetables

This is a good old-fashioned way to prepare chicken for the family.

In a large stew pot, mix all ingredients. Bring to a boil. Reduce heat to a simmer; cover and cook on very low for 50 minutes. Serve with wheat grain noodles.

A Crown of Laurel

Bay leaves, also known as laurel, are originally from the Mediterranean area of the world. They have a strong, woody, and somewhat spicy flavor and are usually sold dried in jars in the spice rack section of the grocery store.

Serves 4

PER SERVING

Calories: 421
GI: Very Low
Carbohydrates: 16 g.
Protein: 39 g.
Fat: 18 g.

1 frying chicken, cut up
1 cup chicken stock
16 pearl onions, peeled
2 large carrots, peeled and
    cut in 1-inch pieces
2 celery stalks, cut in chunks
2 cloves garlic, peeled,
    smashed with the side of
    a knife
1 fennel bulb, trimmed, cut in
    chunks
4 small, bluenose turnips,
    peeled and cut in chunks
1 teaspoon thyme, dried, or
    3 teaspoons fresh
1 teaspoon dried rosemary
2 bay leaves
1 cup dry white wine
2 cups chicken broth
Salt and pepper to taste

Lamb Shanks with White Beans and Carrots

*This is a French bistro and comfort meal that
most people find delicious on a cool evening.*

Serves 4

PER SERVING

Calories: 417
GI: Very Low
Carbohydrates: 44 g.
Protein: 31 g.
Fat: 12 g.

4 lamb shanks, well trimmed
Salt and pepper to taste
1 tablespoon olive oil
1 large yellow onion,
    chopped
4 garlic cloves, minced
1 carrot, peeled and cut in
    chunks
2 tablespoons tomato paste
1 cup dry red wine
1 cup chicken broth
2 bay leaves
¼ cup parsley, chopped
2 13-ounce cans white beans,
    drained

1. Sprinkle the lamb shanks with salt and pepper; brown in the olive oil, adding onion, garlic, and carrot. Cook for 5 minutes. Stir in tomato paste, red wine, chicken broth, bay leaves, and parsley.

2. Cover the pot and simmer for 1 hour. Add white beans and simmer for another 30 minutes.

Not Crazy about Lamb?

When people don't like lamb, it's usually the fat, not the lamb, they dislike. When you prepare roast lamb, stew, or shanks, be sure to remove all of the fat.

Lancaster Lamb Stew

*This dish is reminiscent of a body-warming meal
cooked over a fire on windswept moors.*

1. Sprinkle the lamb with flour, salt, and pepper. Brown it in the butter or margarine. Add all but the potatoes.

2. Cover and simmer for 1 hour. Add the potatoes and cook until tender.

It's All in the Preparations

When preparing lamb, keep in mind that the younger the lamb, the better it tastes.

Serves 4

PER SERVING

Calories: 448
GI: Very Low
Carbohydrates: 38 g.
Protein: 34 g.
Fat: 16 g.

1 pound boneless lamb stew
   meat, well trimmed
1 tablespoon flour
1 teaspoon salt
Pepper to taste
1 tablespoon butter or heart-
   healthy margarine
16 small pearl onions
8 baby carrots
1 tablespoon fresh chervil, or
   1 teaspoon dried
4-inch sprig rosemary leaves,
   stripped from the stem
13-ounce can beef broth
2 ounces Irish whiskey
2 russet potatoes, peeled and
   quartered

Oven-Baked Scrod

*Scrod is light and can stand up to almost any kind of cooking,
from fried for fish and chips to this delicious recipe.*

PER SERVING

Calories: 207
GI: Zero
Carbohydrates: 16 g.
Protein: 31 g.
Fat: 5 g.

⅔ pound scrod filet
Salt and pepper to taste
1 tablespoon lemon juice
2 tablespoons parsley
1 large tomato, thinly sliced
2 tablespoons fine bread
   crumbs
1 tablespoon olive oil
Nonstick spray

1. Preheat the oven to 350°F. Place the fish on an ovenproof pan prepared with nonstick spray.

2. Sprinkle the fish with salt, pepper, lemon juice, and parsley. Arrange the tomato slices on top and sprinkle with bread crumbs. Drizzle olive oil over the top.

3. Bake for 20 to 25 minutes, or until the fish is sizzling and the bread crumbs are brown.

Grilled Pepper Steak

*This recipe combines steak with all the right carbohydrates,
such as those found in onions, peppers, mushrooms, and tomatoes.
You can stack the steak and veggies on a bun or serve on a bed of lettuce.*

Serves 2

PER SERVING

Calories: 284
GI: Zero
Carbohydrates: 9 g.
Protein: 28 g.
Fat: 15 g.

2 cubed steaks (also called
   sandwich steaks)
Salt and pepper to taste
1 teaspoon steak sauce, such
   as A1 or Lea & Perrin's
¼ cup Italian dressing (see
   page 92)
4 frying peppers, cored, seeded,
   and halved, (the thin-
   skinned, light green variety)
1 large portobello mushroom
2 red onions, sliced thick
2 cups lettuce

1. Set the grill on high. Sprinkle the steaks with salt and pepper and spread with steak sauce.

2. Brush the peppers, mushrooms, and onion slices with Italian dressing. Grill steaks for about 4 minutes per side for medium and grill the vegetables until they are slightly charred.

3. Place the steaks on beds of lettuce and pile the veggies on top. Slice the mushroom and arrange with the steaks, peppers, and onions.

Shark Steak with Oranges and Citrus Sauce

*Fresh shark is sweet and tastes especially good when
paired with citrus. Grilled with oranges and served with Caesar salad,
it makes a refreshing lunch or dinner.*

Serves 2

PER SERVING
Calories: 167
GI: Very Low
Carbohydrates: 17 g.
Protein: 18 g.
Fat: 4 g.

⅔ *pound fresh shark filet,
    skin removed*
Salt and pepper to taste
Juice of ½ lemon
Juice of ½ orange
1 tablespoon chili sauce
1 tablespoon sesame seeds
*1 large, thick-skinned orange,
    such as a naval or temple,
    cut crosswise in ½-inch
    slices*
2 sprigs fresh mint leaves
Romaine lettuce

1. Sprinkle the shark with salt and pepper. Whisk the lemon juice, orange juice, and sesame seeds with the chili sauce in a small bowl.

2. Paint the oranges on both sides with the sauce and use the rest on the shark.

3. Place the shark and orange on a hot grill, searing both quickly. Cook for about 3 minutes per side. Serve over lettuce, arranging the orange slices on top of the shark and the mint on top of the orange slices.

Shark Steaks

The most common species of sharks sold as steaks are the mako, blacktip reef shark, and common thresher shark. When purchasing fresh shark steaks, make sure the meat is translucent and does not appear dried out. Also, be sure it does not give off a strong ammonia smell. Flesh should spring back when pressed with your finger.

Chicken in Tomato Sauce

This is another excellent way to get vegetables into your family's diet since the tomato sauce blends well with the flavors of the vegetables. Olives are a tasty addition to this dish.

Serves 4

PER SERVING

Calories: 398
GI: Very Low
Carbohydrates: 11 g.
Protein: 29 g.
Fat: 26 g.

4 chicken legs with thighs
Salt, pepper, and dried thyme
    to taste
1 tablespoon olive oil
2 cloves garlic, chopped
1 large white onion, chopped
1 sweet red pepper, cored and
    chopped
1 stalk celery, chopped
2 okra, finely chopped
1 medium zucchini, chopped
1 teaspoon lemon zest
10 fresh basil leaves, torn
1 teaspoon oregano, dried
2 cups tomato sauce
Optional: 2 slices bacon, fried,
    drained, and crumbled,
    and ¼ cup sliced black or
    green olives for garnish

1. Sprinkle chicken with salt, pepper, and thyme. Heat the olive oil in a large, deep frying pan. Brown the chicken and add onion, garlic, pepper, celery, okra, and zucchini. Stir and cook for 4 minutes.

2. Stir in lemon zest, herbs, and tomato sauce. Cover and simmer for 45 minutes.

3. Garnish, if you like. Serve with couscous or any favorite short pasta.

Basil

Basil is an herb in the mint family and goes particularly well with tomato. Basil is a good choice if you are picking one or two herbs to grow in a small kitchen garden.

Macaroni with Vegetables and Cheese

Everybody loves macaroni and cheese.
Children need calcium and carbohydrates as well as veggies.
Adding some broccoli or spinach makes it fairly healthy.

1. Melt the butter or margarine and stir in the flour. After 3 minutes, whisk in the milk and cheese. Add salt, pepper, sherry, and nutmeg. Set aside.

2. Cook the macaroni according to package directions. Drain and mix with the cheese sauce. Prepare an 8" square pan or an 8" glass pie pan with nonstick spray. Add ½ of the cheese-macaroni mixture. Drop broccoli over the cheese-macaroni mixture.

3. Cover with remaining cheese-macaroni mixture; sprinkle with bread crumbs and grated Parmesan cheese. Bake for 30 minutes in a 325°F oven.

> *Substitute nonfat milk for 2% milk,*
> *use the heart-healthy margarine instead of butter,*
> *and be sure to use low-fat cheese.*

Serves 4

PER SERVING

Calories: 746
GI: Moderate
Carbohydrates: 105 g.
Protein: 32 g.
Fat: 22 g.

1 tablespoon butter or heart-healthy margarine
1 tablespoon flour
2 cups 2% milk
4 ounces sharp Cheddar cheese, grated
Salt and pepper to taste
2 tablespoons dry sherry
¼ teaspoon ground nutmeg
1 pound macaroni
13-ounce package frozen broccoli, thawed and liquid squeezed out
½ cup bread crumbs
½ cup Parmesan cheese, grated
Nonstick spray

Country-Style Pork Ribs

These big, meaty ribs are delicious when properly cooked.
If you don't have a smoker, add some wood chips to your grill,
and if you don't have a grill, use a couple of drops of liquid smoke.
Serve with German-style coleslaw and potato salad.

1. Sprinkle the ribs with salt and pepper, garlic powder, and cayenne pepper. Rub the spices into the meat and bone on both sides. Place them in a turkey roasting pan with the water and liquid smoke on the bottom. Sprinkle with Worcestershire sauce.

2. Set the oven at 225°F. Cover the ribs tightly with aluminum foil. Roast them for 4 to 5 hours. They should be "falling off the bone" tender.

3. Remove foil and brush the ribs with barbeque sauce. Bake for another 15 to 20 minutes or until dark brown.

Liquid Smoke

Liquid smoke is a flavoring for food used to give a smoky, barbequed flavor without the wood chips! It is most often made out of hickory wood, which producers burn to capture and condense the smoke. They filter out impurities in the liquid and bottle the rest.

German-Style Potato Salad

This recipe is exceptionally flavorful and tasty and is wonderful when served with barbequed meats.

1. Peel potatoes and cut into ½-inch slices.

2. Boil the potatoes in salted water to cover, 10 to 15 minutes, or until just softened.

3. Mix the rest of the ingredients in a large bowl. Drain potatoes and add to the dressing immediately. Toss gently to coat. Serve hot or cold.

Serves 4

PER SERVING

Calories: 257
GI: Medium
Carbohydrates: 32 g.
Protein: 4 g.
Fat: 14 g.

2 large Idaho, russet, or Yukon gold potatoes
¼ cup cider vinegar
¼ cup vegetable oil
1 teaspoon salt
1 teaspoon pepper
1 teaspoon sugar
1 teaspoon Hungarian sweet paprika
1 red onion, chopped
2 scallions, chopped
½ cup fresh parsley, chopped

Old-Town Coleslaw

Too much mayonnaise makes coleslaw heavy. Try this Baltimore recipe that is a little lighter on the mayonnaise than traditional slaw recipes.

Mix the dressing in a large bowl. Add the cabbage and onions. Chill for 1 hour and serve.

Serves 4

PER SERVING

Calories: 67
GI: Zero
Carbohydrates: 6 g.
Protein: 1 g.
Fat: 5 g.

¼ cup cider vinegar
1 teaspoon sugar
¼ cup low-fat mayonnaise
¼ teaspoon celery salt
Freshly ground black pepper
¼ teaspoon celery seeds
3 cups shredded cabbage
½ cup red onion, shredded

Sunday Dinner—Roast Chicken

*What could be more traditional than a family dinner of
roast chicken with stuffing, gravy, and delicious vegetables?
Stuffing the chicken with fruit and vegetables helps to lower your GI.*

Serves 4

PER SERVING

Calories: 176
GI: Zero
Carbohydrates: 21 g.
Protein: 3 g.
Fat: 10 g.

2 tablespoons fresh rosemary
 leaves, or 1 tablespoon
 dried
½ lemon, skin and pulp,
 seeded, chopped
3-pound chicken, whole
Salt and pepper to taste
1 teaspoon olive oil
1 apple, peeled, cored, and
 chopped
1 medium red onion,
 chopped
½ fennel bulb, chopped
2 celery stalks, chopped
1 teaspoon thyme leaves
4 prunes, chopped
1 tablespoon orange peel
2 ounces walnuts, chopped
1 cup chicken broth

1. Mix the rosemary and lemon pulp and sprinkle the chicken with salt and pepper. Push the lemon and rosemary under the skin of the chicken, working it right down into the thigh.

2. Heat the olive oil and sauté the apple, onion, fennel, celery, thyme, prunes, and orange peel for 10 minutes. Add the walnuts at the end. When cool enough to handle, stuff the chicken. Close the openings at neck and tail with small skewers.

3. Roast the chicken for 90 minutes at 350°F; baste every 15 minutes with the chicken broth.

Black Bean Chili with Beef and Corn

This will give your family a meal with real punch, staying power, and nutrition.

1. In a large, ovenproof casserole, heat the oil over medium flame. Brown the beef. Move to one side of the casserole dish and sauté the vegetables for 5 minutes. Stir in the cumin and herbs and mix well.

2. Preheat oven to 340°F. Stir in the corn, black beans, tomatoes, salt, and pepper. Sprinkle with lime juice. Stir to mix.

3. Spread the top with cheese and bake for 30 minutes, or until hot and bubbling. Serve with corn bread or tortillas.

Legumes

Beans are legumes, as are other foods such as lentils, peas, soybeans, and peanuts. Not only are legumes good for farmers to produce because their roots produce nitrogen, which fertilizes land, but they are delicious and full of healthy protein for you!

Serves 4

PER SERVING

Calories: 429
GI: Low
Carbohydrates: 69 g.
Protein: 23 g.
Fat: 13 g.

---

2 tablespoons olive or other cooking oil
½ pound ground beef
1 large red onion, chopped
2 cloves garlic, minced
1 large sweet red bell pepper, cored, seeded, and chopped
1 small hot pepper, cored, seeded, and minced
1 teaspoon ground cumin
1 teaspoon dried cilantro or parsley (fresh is better)
8 ounces frozen corn niblets
2 13-ounce cans black beans, drained
1 cup crushed tomatoes (canned is fine)
Salt and pepper to taste
Juice of ½ lime
2 ounces Monterey Jack cheese, shredded

Pot Roast with Vegetables and Gravy

*As a family dinner, this can't be beat. The leftovers can be reheated
with gravy and served over noodles or toast for a quick lunch or supper.*

Serves 6

PER SERVING

Calories: 590
GI: Very Low
Carbohydrates: 24 g.
Protein: 67 g.
Fat: 24 g.

2 tablespoons canola oil
Salt and pepper to taste
3 pounds beef bottom round
    roast, trimmed of fat
4 sweet medium onions,
    chopped
4 cloves garlic, chopped
4 carrots, peeled and
    chopped
4 celery stalks, chopped
8 small bluenose turnips,
    peeled and chopped
1 inch gingerroot, peeled and
    minced
13-ounce can beef broth
½ cup dry red wine
Wondra flour to thicken

1. Brown the beef at medium-high heat in a large pot and set aside; add the vegetables to the pot and cook, stirring until wilted. Return the beef to the pot and add the rest of the ingredients. Cover and cook over very low heat for 3 hours.

2. To serve, slice the beef across, not with, the grain. Serve surrounded by vegetables and place the gravy on the side or over the top.

> *You can lower the fat of this recipe by reducing
> the amount of meat you use and by browning
> the meat in cooking spray instead of oil.*

Chapter 14

Holiday Fare: Drinks and Meals

Makes 80 ounces,
20 servings

Per Serving

Calories: 176
GI: Low
Carbohydrates: 15 g.
Protein: 0 g.
Fat: 0 g.

2 quarts dry red wine
1 cup cognac
1 cup orange Curacao
½ cup sugar, or to taste
10 cloves
4 cinnamon sticks
1 orange, sliced
1 lemon, sliced

Hot Mulled Wine

This is festive on a cold winter evening and makes a large enough batch for entertaining. Sip in front of the fireplace to warm yourself from the inside out!

Eight hours before serving place all ingredients in a nonreactive pot and marinate. When ready to serve, bring to a boil, reduce heat, and serve warm.

Makes 2 drinks

Per Serving

Calories: 93
GI: Low
Carbohydrates: 9 g.
Protein: 0 g.
Fat: 0 g.

1 ounce Lemon-flavored
   vodka (like Absolute
   Citron)
2 ounces hard cider
2 ounces plain cider
1 ounce fresh lime juice

Country Cousin

With all the buzz about the cosmopolitan cocktail,
you might like to try a country version.

Shake all ingredients with ice and pour into chilled cocktail glasses.

Vita-C

Restoratives are part of alcoholic history. During the holidays, you sometimes need a boost. This drink is sure to pep you up!

In a pitcher filled with ice, stir the first three ingredients. Add the champagne and serve.

Makes 4 drinks, 5 ounces each

PER SERVING (WITH CHAMPAGNE)

Calories: 130
GI: High
Carbohydrates: 17 g.
Protein: 1 g.
Fat: 0 g.

*8 ounces fresh orange juice
2 ounces orange Curacao
2 ounces freshly squeezed lemon juice
Optional: 1 tablespoon sugar syrup
8 ounces brut champagne or sparkling water*

Breath o' Christmas

When you are using acidic ingredients, it is smart to use enamel-coated, stainless steel, or well-seasoned wrought iron pots and pans. Do not use tin or aluminum since the acid will react with those metals. Acids include tomatoes, citrus, wine, and spirits.

Make the hot cocoa according to package directions. Add the Crème de Menthe. Top with cream whipped with the vanilla and sugar.

You may substitute whole or 2% milk for heavy cream in this drink.

Makes 1 serving

PER SERVING

Calories: 426
GI: Moderate
Carbohydrates: 28 g.
Protein: 5 g.
Fat: 29 g.

*6 ounces hot cocoa
1 ounce Crème de Menthe
¼ cup heavy cream
½ teaspoon vanilla
½ teaspoon confectioners' sugar*

Mocha Cream Irish Coffee

*An after dinner drink, sipped slowly with some great conversation
is an excellent ending to the evening's pleasures. This drink is so rich
that a little goes a long way.*

In a saucepan, mix all ingredients together and stir to dissolve sugar.
Serve hot.

> *In this recipe, you can substitute whole
> or 2% milk for cream.*

Makes 1 cup

PER SERVING

Calories: 235
GI: Moderate
Carbohydrates: 8 g.
Protein: 3 g.
Fat: 17 g.

½ cup hot cocoa
2 ounces hot coffee
*1 teaspoon sugar substitute,
  or to taste*
1 ounce heavy cream
1 ounce Irish whiskey
Sprinkle of cinnamon on top

Hot Buttered Rum

*A rich, sweet drink like hot buttered rum is great for dessert. There are hundreds
of recipes for hot buttered rum—this is one of the best! Serve in coffee mugs.*

Using a fork, mix the brown sugar, butter, and lemon juice together with
the nutmeg and rum. When well mixed, add the boiling water. Serve
immediately.

Makes 1 drink

PER SERVING

Calories: 282
GI: Moderate
Carbohydrates: 13 g.
Protein: 0 g.
Fat: 12 g.

1 tablespoon brown sugar
1 tablespoon unsalted butter
1 teaspoon lemon juice
1 pinch nutmeg
2 ounces rum
4 ounces boiling water

Pink Champagne Cocktail

Celebrate the holidays with this great cocktail! It will whet your appetite and will not spoil your dinner like sweeter dessert drinks.

Mix the Chambord and Curacao in a flute glass. Add the champagne. Toast!

Makes 1 serving

PER SERVING

Calories: 314
GI: Moderate
Carbohydrates: 33 g.
Protein: 0 g.
Fat: 0 g.

1 ounce Chambord (raspberry liqueur)
1 ounce orange Curacao
4 ounces dry brut champagne

Mulled, Spiced Cider

This is festive for nondrinkers and kids.
Serve nice and hot on a chilly fall day or winter's night.

Mix all ingredients together, heat, and serve.

Makes 1 quart, 8 servings

**PER SERVING
(4 OUNCES)**

Calories: 112
GI: Moderate
Carbohydrates: 30 g.
Protein: 0 g.
Fat: 0 g.

28 ounces cider
Juice of 1 lemon
1 orange, sliced thinly and seeded
10 whole cloves
2 cinnamon sticks
½ teaspoon allspice, not ground

Frozen Watermelon and Vodka Balls

This is a grownup treat for a hot Fourth of July!

Serves 10

PER SERVING
(8 OUNCES)

Calories: 58
GI: High
Carbohydrates: 6 g.
Protein: 1 g.
Fat: 0 g.

5 cups watermelon balls, seedless
5 ounces vodka
10 mint leaves for garnish

1. Use a melon baller to scoop balls of watermelon. Place the watermelon balls in a plastic container and pour the vodka over them. Cover and freeze for 30 minutes.

2. Turn container upside down to spread vodka and freeze for another 30 minutes. Serve in champagne flutes and top each with a mint leaf.

French Punch

Special occasions held on a warm afternoon are enhanced by a punch.
When preparing for a party, put 2 cups of water into a
1-quart plastic container. Fill the container with strawberries,
sliced peaches, and lemons, limes, or oranges.
Freeze the night before and float in your punchbowl for the party.

Serves 15

PER SERVING
(5 OUNCES)

Calories: 119
GI: Moderate
Carbohydrates: 1 g.
Protein: 0 g.
Fat: 0 g.

2 cups cognac, chilled
1 28-ounce bottle dry brut champagne, chilled
1 4-ounce can frozen pink lemonade
1 25-ounce bottle lemon-flavored Perrier water, chilled
1 quart container frozen water with strawberries, sliced peaches, and sliced lemons, limes, or oranges

Mix all ingredients together just before serving and float the ice to keep punch chilled.

Raw Oysters on the Half Shell with Mignonette Sauce

This is a wonderful holiday appetizer. You can make the mignonette sauce in advance. Oysters should be served the day they are opened. Tell your fishmonger not to rinse off the liquor (natural juice). The oyster liquor is full of great flavor!

Place the shallots, lemon juice, parsley, salt, and pepper in the blender. On low speed, slowly add the olive oil. Spoon over the oysters.

Serves 2

PER SERVING

Calories: 155
GI: Zero
Carbohydrates: 7 g.
Protein: 7 g.
Fat: 11 g.

12 raw oysters, on the half shell, resting on a bed of ice
2 shallots, minced
1 tablespoon lemon juice
1 tablespoon Italian parsley, chopped
Salt and pepper to taste
½ cup extra-virgin olive oil

Broiled Quail with Claret Glaze

Quail, which is a small game bird in the pheasant family, makes a festive winter dish.

1. Boil down the wine and orange juice, reducing to 1 cup.

2. Preheat the broiler to 400°F. Mix the olive oil, lemon juice, salt, and pepper and brush it on both sides of the quail. Broil, inside up, for 5 minutes; brush both sides with wine mixture and turn. Broil for another 10 minutes, brushing every few minutes with the wine/orange juice mixture.

Serves 4

PER SERVING

Calories: 674
GI: Low
Carbohydrates: 14 g.
Protein: 50 g.
Fat: 30 g.

2 cups claret or port wine
1 teaspoon concentrated orange juice
8 quail, about 4 ounces each, split open at the back
2 teaspoons olive oil
1 tablespoon lemon juice
Salt and pepper to taste

Baked Oysters with Shrimp Stuffing

This recipe is perfect for those who would rather eat their oysters cooked. Always taste the liquor for saltiness. Some oysters are very salty; some are not. This is an easy recipe for a romantic dinner or you can just add to it for a party.

Serves 2

PER SERVING

Calories: 222
GI: Low
Carbohydrates: 20 g.
Protein: 16 g.
Fat: 10 g.

1 teaspoon butter
2 shallots, chopped
2 slices bacon, fried and
   crumbled
1 tablespoon lemon juice
2 slices stale white bread,
   crumbled
4 medium shrimp, raw,
   peeled, deveined, and
   chopped
Salt, if necessary
Plenty of freshly ground
   pepper
8 raw oysters, on the half
   shell, liquor reserved

1. Set oven at 425°F. Melt the butter; add shallots and sauté for 5 minutes on medium heat. Add the crumbled bacon and lemon juice.

2. Stir in the bread crumbs and mix in the oyster liquor. Taste for saltiness, add shrimp, and grind on pepper.

3. Divide the bread and shrimp mixture among the oysters. Bake for 12 to 15 minutes, or until the oysters are bubbling and the topping is well browned.

Substitute vegetarian bacon for regular bacon and replace butter with olive oil.

Regional Oysters

Depending on where they come from, oysters can have different flavors. Some oysters are extremely sweet and light in flavor. Some Pacific Coast oysters taste metallic, and oysters from certain estuaries have a distinctly swampy flavor. Oysters from Long Island Sound are exported to Japan and France and are very sweet tasting.

Holiday Chestnut Soup

This is an elegant starter for a holiday meal.

1. Preheat oven to 450°F. Make a cut in the side of each chestnut and bake on a sheet until the edges of the cut peel back and the nut meat is soft, about 15 to 20 minutes. Peel when cool.

2. In a large soup kettle, melt the butter and sauté the shallots and garlic until soft, about 10 minutes. Add nutmeg and flour, stirring to blend.

3. Whisk in the beef broth. Place chestnuts and 2 cups of the liquid mixture in the blender and purée. Return to the kettle and whisk to blend.

4. Cover and simmer over low heat for 20 minutes. Whisk in the cream; taste and adjust salt and pepper. Serve hot with a sprig of watercress on each bowl of soup.

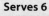 *Substitute olive oil for butter in this soup to reduce calories.*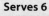

Serves 6

PER SERVING

Calories: 341
GI: Moderate
Carbohydrates: 44 g.
Protein: 3 g.
Fat: 18 g.

---

1 tablespoon butter, unsalted
4 shallots, minced
1 clove garlic, minced
¼ teaspoon nutmeg
1 tablespoon Wondra quick-
    blending flour
2 13-ounce cans beef broth,
    low-salt
1 pound chestnuts
1 cup whipping cream
Salt and pepper to taste
Garnish of ½ cup stemmed,
    loosely packed watercress

Duck Breasts Sautéed with Rum-Raisin Sauce

This is a different and delectable take on two holiday classics.
Sweet rum-raisin sauce is often used in desserts—this one is not so sweet.

Serves 4

PER SERVING

Calories: 215
GI: Moderate
Carbohydrates: 18 g.
Protein: 14 g.
Fat: 8 g.

2 duck breasts, about ½
    pound each, skinless and
    boneless
Salt and pepper to taste
2 tablespoons flour
¼ teaspoon ground nutmeg
¼ teaspoon ground cloves
1 tablespoon extra-virgin
    olive oil
½ cup chicken broth
2 tablespoons golden rum
½ cup golden raisins (sultana)
Extra salt and pepper, to taste
1 teaspoon Wondra quick-
    blending flour
¼ cup light cream

1. Roll the duck breasts in a mixture of salt, pepper, flour, nutmeg, and cloves. Sauté in olive oil over medium heat until brown on both sides. Set aside, covered with aluminum foil on a warm platter.

2. To the pan in which the duck was cooked, add chicken broth and rum. Bring to a boil. Add raisins, salt, pepper, and flour. Turn the heat down and simmer for 5 minutes. Add cream and pour over duck breasts.

Duck? Delicious!

While most people believe duck meat to be extremely fattening, it is the skin that is the culprit and not the meat of the duck. Duck meat is actually very lean when prepared without the skin and contains large amounts of protein and iron.

Venison with Chestnut Purée and Spiced Currant Jelly

The recipes for Chestnut Purée and Spiced Currant Jelly are found on page 224.
Venison is tender and delicious, a light, grass-fed meat.
Farm-raised venison can be ordered on the Internet.

1. Using a mortar and pestle, mash the garlic, Worcestershire sauce, and pepper together. Spread on the venison and let stand for 30 minutes to permeate the medallions.

2. In a frying pan set over medium heat, warm the olive oil and sauté the venison for 6 minutes per side.

3. Place on a warm platter and loosely cover. Pour the beef broth and wine into the pan and bring to a boil. Pour sauce over the venison.

4. Sprinkle with parsley and serve.

Serves 4

PER SERVING
(VENISON ALONE)

Calories: 172
GI: Zero
Carbohydrates: 2 g.
Protein: 6 g.
Fat: 7 g.

2 cloves garlic, minced
1 tablespoon Worcestershire
  sauce
½ teaspoon freshly ground
  black pepper
4 medallions of venison,
  about ⅓ pound each
1 tablespoon olive oil
¼ cup beef broth
¼ cup dry red wine
¼ cup stemmed, loosely
  packed fresh parsley,
  chopped

Chestnut Purée

*This is just as wonderful with venison as with turkey, game hens, or duck.
If you use chestnuts from a can or a jar, you will save a great deal of time.*

Purée all ingredients in a blender or food processor. Warm over low heat and serve.

Makes 1 cup, 8 servings

**PER SERVING
(2 TABLESPOONS)**

Calories: 79
GI: Moderate
Carbohydrates: 16 g.
Protein: 2 g.
Fat: 2 g.

*8 ounces chestnuts, shelled
Salt and pepper to taste
Pinch nutmeg
½ cup whole milk or light
    cream*

Spiced Currant Jelly

*This is another excellent condiment, good anytime
to dress up meat, game, or poultry.*

Put all ingredients in a saucepan. Warm over low heat and simmer for 3 minutes. Pour into a bowl and serve.

Makes 1 cup, 8 servings

**PER SERVING
(2 TABLESPOONS)**

Calories: 102
GI: High
Carbohydrates: 26 g.
Protein: 0 g.
Fat: 0 g.

*1 cup currant jelly
4 whole cloves
½-inch slice orange with peel,
    seeded and chopped
½ cinnamon stick*

Winter Root Vegetable Soufflé

*This recipe puts to good use all of the wonderful
root vegetables available in the winter months and provides
an alternative to simply mashing them with butter.*

Serves 4

PER SERVING

Calories: 200
GI: High
Carbohydrates: 28 g.
Protein: 11 g.
Fat: 6 g.

½ large Vidalia onion, cut in
    big chunks
2 carrots, peeled and
    chopped
2 parsnips, peeled and
    chopped
2 baby turnips, peeled and
    cut in pieces
1 teaspoon salt, in water for
    boiling vegetables
4 eggs, separated, whites
    reserved
1 teaspoon dried sage
2 tablespoons parsley,
    chopped, fresh only
1 tablespoon flour
½ teaspoon Tabasco sauce, or
    to taste
½ cup 2% milk
Nonstick spray

1. Set oven on 400°F. Place the cleaned vegetables in a pot of cold, salted water to cover. Bring to a boil; reduce heat and simmer until the veggies are very tender when pierced with a fork.

2. Drain the vegetables and cool slightly. Place in the blender and purée. With the blender running on medium speed, add the egg yolks, one at a time. Then add the sage, parsley, flour, Tabasco sauce, and milk. Pour into a bowl.

3. Prepare a 2-quart soufflé dish with nonstick spray. Beat the egg whites until stiff. Fold the egg whites into the purée. Pour into the soufflé dish.

4. Bake the soufflé for 20 minutes at 400°F. Reduce heat to 350°F and bake for 20 minutes more. Don't worry if your soufflé flops just before serving; it will still be light and delicious.

 You can substitute nonfat milk for 2% milk when making this soufflé.

Soufflé Tip

It's okay to have a soufflé flop, especially in the case of cheese and vegetable soufflés. A dessert soufflé should never fall. If, as directed, you start the soufflé with the oven on 400°F and then reduce the temperature, you are more likely to produce a high soufflé!

Whole Roast Filet Mignon with Mustard Cream Sauce (Hot)

Filet mignon is equally good served hot, cold, or at room temperature. If you are serving buffet style, go for room temperature.

Serves 14

PER SERVING
(SAUCE NOT INCLUDED)

Calories: 416
GI: Low
Carbohydrates: 8 g.
Protein: 46 g.
Fat: 15 g.

5 pound filet mignon, fat and
    skin removed
Salt and pepper
2 cloves minced garlic,
    mashed in a press
½ cup beef broth
¼ cup dry red wine
10 tiny new potatoes, skin on,
    cut in halves
15 baby carrots
25 pearl onions
Mustard Cream Sauce (Hot)
    (see page 237)

1. Preheat the oven to 400°F. Spread the salt, pepper, and garlic on the filet mignon. Place in a roasting pan with red wine and beef broth and roast for 10 minutes. Reduce heat to 350°F and add the vegetables. Baste every 5 minutes.

2. Roast the filet mignon for another 20 minutes for medium rare. Continue basting, turning the vegetables every 8 to 10 minutes.

3. Let the meat rest. Serve sliced and surrounded with potatoes, vegetables, and Mustard Cream Sauce (Hot).

Meat Temperatures

Remember that meat cooked in the oven, on the grill, or in a sauté pan continues to rise another 5-plus degrees after it is removed from the heat source. So if overcooking has been a problem, take your meat off the heat sooner, or 5 degrees short of the doneness temperature desired.

Country Ham

A country ham is a beautiful thing! Depending on where they come from, country hams are smoked or salt cured. Both are improved by soaking.

1. Prepare the ham by removing skin and most of the fat, leaving ¼ inch of fat.

2. Soak ham in water to cover with bay leaves, brown sugar, cloves, peppercorns, and coriander seeds for 30 hours.

3. Preheat the oven to 300°F. Pat the ham dry and place in a roasting pan. Spread with the rest of the brown sugar, mixed with the mustard and cloves.

4. Bake for 3-½ hours, basting with the apple cider. You can degrease the pan juices and use the apple cider as a sauce; otherwise, serve with applesauce.

Serves 20

PER SERVING (NOT INCLUDING APPLE CIDER)

Calories: 403
GI: Low
Carbohydrates: 0 g.
Protein: 51 g.
Fat: 21 g.

10-pound country ham, bone in
Water to cover
10 bay leaves
1 pound brown sugar
20 whole cloves, bruised
25 peppercorns, bruised
10 coriander seeds, bruised
½ cup brown sugar
2 tablespoons dark mustard
½ teaspoon powdered cloves
1-½ cups apple cider

Cranberry Ring with Walnut, Celeriac, Dried Cranberry, and Apple Salad

This is another old-fashioned dish, adapted for modern tables.

Serves 8

PER SERVING

Calories: 315
GI: Low
Carbohydrates: 38 g.
Protein: 5 g.
Fat: 18 g.

2 envelopes unflavored
    gelatin
2 cups cranberry juice
    cocktail, sugar-free,
    heated
1 teaspoon Tabasco sauce
1 cup 100% cranberry juice,
    sugar-free, cold
¼ cup orange juice
2 tart apples, peeled, cored,
    and chopped
½ cup walnuts, toasted,
    chopped
1 whole celeriac root, peeled
    and grated
½ cup dried cranberries
1 cup low-fat mayonnaise
¼ cup white wine vinegar

1. Place the gelatin in the bowl of the blender. Cover with ¼ cup of cold cranberry juice and allow to bloom for 5 minutes, expanding and softening. With the blender running on medium speed, add the hot cranberry juice cocktail, Tabasco sauce, the remaining cold cranberry juice, and orange juice. Pour into a 1-½ quart ring mold.

2. Add one apple. Refrigerate until set, about 2 hours.

3. Make the salad by mixing the walnuts, celeriac, dried cranberries and the second apple, vinegar, and mayonnaise together. When ready to serve, fill the ring and surround it with the salad.

Wild Rice Casserole with Hazelnuts and Dried Apricots

This rice dish has a hint of fruity sweetness from the apricots that will make it a standout side dish at your holiday table.

1. Bring the water to a boil; add the wild rice and salt. Reduce heat; cover and simmer for 1 hour or until grains are fully opened.

2. Sauté the onion in the butter. In a separate bowl, cover the apricots with chicken broth and allow to expand for 30 minutes. When the rice is fully cooked, place in a casserole dish. Add the sautéed onions, apricots soaked in broth, nuts, baked ham, and pepper.

3. Dot with 2 teaspoons butter and bake for 15 minutes at 250°F, letting the flavors blend.

> ♥ Substitute heart-healthy margarine or olive oil for butter in this casserole. ♥

Wild Rice Basics

When cooking wild rice, always use more liquid than the recipe on the box suggests. Wild rice should fully bloom, not be tiny spikes when cooked.

Serves 8

PER SERVING

Calories: 183
GI: Moderate
Carbohydrates: 22 g.
Protein: 6 g.
Fat: 10 g.

---

4 cups water
1 cup wild rice
1 teaspoon salt, or to taste
1 tablespoon butter
½ sweet onion, such as Vidalia, chopped
1 cup dried apricots, cut in pieces
1 cup chicken broth
½ cup hazelnuts, toasted
½ cup baked ham, chopped fine
Freshly ground black pepper to taste

Fresh Corn Stuffing for Poultry, Fish, or Game

Stuffing can be piled on top of a dish instead of being stuffed into meat.
This dish is exceptional, a remembrance of the first Thanksgiving
and the Native American's gift of corn to the starving Pilgrims.

1. Melt the butter or margarine in a pan over medium heat. Sauté the onions and celery for 5 to 7 minutes.

2. Add the broth, herbs, and spices. Mix well and add the cornbread stuffing, corn, and milk. Use with any holiday entrée!

> *To lower the fat and calories of this recipe,*
> *substitute heart-healthy margarine or olive oil*
> *for butter and replace 2% milk with nonfat milk.*

chapter 15
Dressings and Sauces

Country Barbecue Sauce

*You can change the flavor of this sauce by adding a
chopped lemon, orange juice, or lime juice.*

Makes 1 quart, 8 servings

**PER SERVING
(4 OUNCES)**

Calories: 118
GI: Very Low
Carbohydrates: 18 g.
Protein: 3 g.
Fat: 4 g.

*2 large yellow onions,
    chopped
4 cloves garlic, chopped
2 sweet red peppers, cored,
    seeded, and chopped
2 serrano chili peppers, cored,
    seeded, and minced
    (optional)
2 tablespoons olive oil
1 teaspoon salt, or to taste
2 teaspoons black pepper
1 teaspoon Tabasco sauce, or
    to taste
2 ounces cider vinegar
2 tablespoons Dijon-style
    prepared mustard
28-ounce can tomato purée
2 tablespoons molasses
1 teaspoon liquid smoke
4 whole cloves
1 cinnamon stick
1 teaspoon hot paprika
1 tablespoon sweet paprika*

1. In a large soup pot, sauté the garlic, onions, and peppers in olive oil. Stirring constantly, add the rest of the ingredients. Bring to a boil. Reduce heat.

2. Cover the pot and simmer for 2 hours. If you don't like the texture, purée in the blender.

Sweet, Spicy, or Both

The amount of heat you add to barbeque sauce is a matter of personal taste, as is the amount of sweetness. Some people prefer the flavor of honey over molasses; others use brown sugar. Experiment!

Yogurt and Herb (Ranch)

This is delicious with vegetables.

Whisk all ingredients together and serve.

Makes 1 cup, 8 servings

**PER SERVING
(2 TABLESPOONS)**

Calories: 17
GI: Very Low
Carbohydrates: 2 g.
Protein: 1 g.
Fat: 0 g.

7 ounces low-fat yogurt
2 tablespoons lemon juice
2 tablespoons chives,
    chopped
½ teaspoon celery salt
½ teaspoon garlic powder
2 drops Tabasco sauce, or to
    taste

Lemon Pepper Dressing

*Peppercorns and chilies offer different flavors in cooking.
Peppercorns are dried berries, and chilies are the hot fruit of a plant
and have spicy seeds. This recipe is a wonderful marriage of pepper flavors.
Use it with grilled vegetables, as well as on salads.*

Whisk all ingredients together and serve with chicken, salad, or cold
meats.

Makes 1 cup, 8 servings

**PER SERVING
(1 OUNCE)**

Calories: 81
GI: Zero
Carbohydrates: 2 g.
Protein: 0 g.
Fat: 8 g.

7 ounces low-fat mayonnaise
Juice and minced rind of ½
    lemon
1 teaspoon Dijon-style
    mustard
1 teaspoon black pepper,
    freshly ground
½ teaspoon white pepper
½ teaspoon red pepper flakes
Salt to taste
¼ teaspoon anchovy paste

Caesar Dressing

True Caesar salad dressing has a touch of anchovy, lemon, and mustard.

**PER SERVING
(1 OUNCE)**

Calories: 83
GI: Zero
Carbohydrates: 0 g.
Protein: 2 g.
Fat: 9 g.

1. In the blender, blend the vinegar, egg, garlic, and lemon juice until puréed. Add the mustard, anchovy paste, salt, pepper, and cheese.

2. With the blender running on medium speed, slowly pour in the olive oil in a thin stream. Garnish with fresh parsley to taste.

¼ cup red wine vinegar
1 raw (pasteurized) egg
1 clove garlic, mashed
1 tablespoon lemon juice
½ teaspoon dry English
      mustard
½ inch anchovy paste
Salt and pepper to taste
¼ cup Parmesan cheese,
      freshly grated
¾ cup olive oil
Garnish of parsley to taste

Which Olive Oil is Best?

Extra-virgin olive oil comes from the first pressing of the olives, has the most intense flavor, and is the most expensive. Use this for salads and for dressings and dips. Virgin olive oil is from the second pressing. Less expensive than extra-virgin, it can be used for the same purposes. "Olive oil" indicates that it is from the last pressing; this is the oil used for cooking since it does not burn as easily at high temperatures.

Hollandaise Sauce

*If you make Hollandaise sauce in the blender or
food processor, your sauce will not curdle.*

Makes ¾ cup, 6 servings

**Per Serving
(1 ounce)**

Calories: 161
GI: Zero
Carbohydrates: 0 g.
Protein: 2 g.
Fat: 17 g.

---

*4 ounces sweet unsalted
    butter
1 whole egg
1 egg yolk
¼ teaspoon dry mustard
Juice of ½ lemon
⅛ teaspoon cayenne pepper
Salt to taste*

1. Melt the butter over very low heat. While the butter is melting, blend all but the salt in the blender or food processor.

2. With the blender running on medium speed, slowly add the butter, a little at a time. Return the sauce to a low heat and whisk until thickened. Add salt and serve immediately.

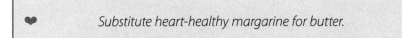

Substitute heart-healthy margarine for butter.

Bernaise Sauce and Sauce Maltaise

If you substitute white wine vinegar for lemon juice and add chives in this recipe, you will have Bernaise Sauce, a classic for steaks. If you substitute orange juice for lemon juice, you'll have Sauce Maltaise, which is delicious with vegetables.

Horseradish Sauce

This is a classic with corned beef. It can be used for hot or cold meats, fish, or seafood. When you see rosy horseradish in the supermarket, try it. Rosy horseradish is colored and slightly sweetened with beet juice.

Using a fork, mix all ingredients together in a bowl and serve.

Makes 1 cup, 8 servings

Per Serving (1 ounce)

Calories: 32
GI: Very Low
Carbohydrates: 1 g.
Protein: 0 g.
Fat: 3 g.

1 cup low-fat sour cream
1 tablespoon prepared horseradish
1 tablespoon lemon juice
Salt and freshly ground black pepper to taste

Sweet and Sour Dressing

You can use this as a dressing for salad, especially Asian noodle salads, or hot noodles. You can also use it on pork, chicken, or beef.

Whisk all ingredients together over low heat until well blended and serve.

Makes ½ cup, 8 servings

Per Serving (1 tablespoon)

Calories: 22
GI: Low
Carbohydrates: 4 g.
Protein: 0 g.
Fat: 1 g.

3 ounces soy sauce
1 teaspoon Asian sesame seed oil
1 teaspoon fresh ginger, minced
1 tablespoon maple syrup or honey
1 tablespoon concentrated orange juice
1 tablespoon apricot preserves or jam
1 clove garlic, minced
1 teaspoon Tabasco sauce, or to taste

Mustard Cream Sauce (Hot)

This is a perfect complement to chicken, goose, duck, or veal.

1. Heat the olive oil over medium flame. Add the shallots and garlic; sauté for 5 minutes or until soft. Whisk in the flour and cook for another 2 to 3 minutes. Whisk in the chicken broth, vermouth, and mustard.

2. Bring the sauce to a boil. Whisk in the cream and turn off heat. Taste for salt and pepper and add accordingly.

Serves 4

Per Serving (2 ounces)

Calories: 111
GI: Very Low
Carbohydrates: 1 g.
Protein: 0 g.
Fat: 0 g.

2 tablespoons olive oil
2 shallots, minced
1 clove garlic, minced
1 teaspoon flour
⅔ cup chicken broth
1 ounce dry vermouth
1 tablespoon Dijon-style mustard, prepared
2 ounces heavy cream
Salt and pepper to taste

Egg and Parsley Sauce (Hot)

When you prepare poached salmon, serve smoked salmon for brunch, or want to make a special dish of chicken breasts, try this sauce.

1. Heat the olive oil or butter over medium flame. Sauté the shallots for 6 to 8 minutes, until softened. Blend in the flour. Cook for 2 minutes.

2. Whisk in the cream. Bring to a scald; add hard-boiled egg, salt, pepper, and spices. Serve immediately.

Makes 1 cup, 8 servings

Per Serving (1 ounce)

Calories: 119
GI: Very Low
Carbohydrates: 2 g.
Protein: 1 g.
Fat: 13 g.

1 tablespoon olive oil
4 shallots, minced
1 tablespoon Wondra quick-blending flour
¼ cup stemmed, loosely packed fresh Italian flat-leaf parsley, chopped
1 cup light cream, warmed
1 hard-boiled egg
Salt and pepper to taste
Pinch nutmeg

Aioli

Aioli is a basic French mayonnaise used throughout the Mediterranean.
It's loaded with garlic and can have a variety of different herbs.
You can add tomatoes and spices.

Makes 1 cup, 16 servings

PER SERVING
(1 TABLESPOON)

Calories: 99
GI: Zero
Carbohydrates: 0 g.
Protein: 1 g.
Fat: 12 g.

2 pasteurized eggs, at room temperature
1 teaspoon lemon juice
1 teaspoon white wine vinegar
½ teaspoon Dijon-style mustard
4 cloves garlic, or to taste
¾ cup olive oil
Choice of: ½ teaspoon oregano, tarragon, or rosemary
Salt and pepper to taste

1. Place the eggs, lemon juice, vinegar, mustard, and garlic in the blender.

2. Add the olive oil a little at a time. When the mixture is creamy, taste; add herbs, salt, and pepper. Pulse to blend; store in the refrigerator or serve.

Storing Aioli

Aioli will keep in the refrigerator for a day or two, but it's best made and used the same day.

Hot Mustard Aioli

Use the Aioli recipe (see facing page) with the following changes.
It is wonderful on cold lamb or roast beef.

1. Place all ingredients but the olive oil, salt, and pepper sauce in the blender. Add the olive oil a few drops at a time.

2. When the aioli is thick, add salt and pepper sauce and blend. Serve or store in the refrigerator.

Mustard

Recipes often call for Dijon mustard or Dijon-style mustard (for example, Grey Poupon). German-style mustards can often be interchanged with Dijon. They are all robust.

Makes 1 cup, 16 servings

**PER SERVING
(1 TABLESPOON)**

Calories: 100
GI: Zero
Carbohydrates: 0 g.
Protein: 1 g.
Fat: 12 g.

---

2 pasteurized eggs, at room
    temperature
1 teaspoon lemon juice
1 teaspoon white wine
    vinegar
1 tablespoon prepared,
    Dijon-style mustard
4 garlic cloves, or to taste
Choice of: ½ teaspoon
    oregano, tarragon, or
    rosemary
¾ cup olive oil
Salt to taste
Hot red pepper sauce to taste

Makes 1 cup, 16 servings

**PER SERVING
(1 TABLESPOON)**

Calories: 12
GI: Very Low
Carbohydrates: 5 g.
Protein: 0 g.
Fat: 0 g.

1 mango, peeled and diced
½ cup cranberries, coarsely
     ground in the food
     processor or blender
½ cup sugar substitute
1 tablespoon lemon juice
1 hot chili, cored, seeded, and
     chopped
½ teaspoon salt
1 tablespoon orange peel, fresh

Makes 1 cup, 8 servings

**PER SERVING
(2 TABLESPOONS)**

Calories: 85
GI: Very Low
Carbohydrates: 0 g.
Protein: 1 g.
Fat: 5 g.

⅔ cup green olives, pitted
     and chopped
½ cup fresh parsley
Juice of ½ lemon
Rind of ½ lemon, minced
1 tablespoon chives, minced,
     fresh only
1 cup cream cheese, at room
     temperature
Freshly ground black pepper
     to taste

Mango-Cranberry Salsa

Try this for a change at Thanksgiving or on any poultry or pork.

Mix all ingredients together the day before you plan to serve the salsa.
Cover and refrigerate.

Green Olive Sauce

*This is a wonderful garnish or spread for a good hot Tuscan bread.
There is no salt in this recipe because the olives are very salty.*

Mix all ingredients together. Chill for 2 hours. Serve at room temperature.

*You can substitute low-fat cream cheese
for regular cream cheese in this spread.*

Grilled Peach Chutney

Grilled fruit is wonderful with any number of meats, poultry, or fish.
Grilled peach chutney is sublime!

1. Grill the peaches, cut side down, over low flame until they are soft but not falling apart, about 5 minutes.

2. Cool them and then slip off the skins. Using a knife, cut them into chunks and place in a bowl. This method retains the juice and some texture.

3. Mix the rest of the ingredients into the bowl with the peaches. Cool, cover, and refrigerate until ready to serve. Warm just before serving.

Makes 2 cups, 16 servings

PER SERVING
(2 TABLESPOONS)

Calories: 45
GI: Very Low
Carbohydrates: 12 g.
Protein: 0 g.
Fat: 0 g.

6 medium-sized freestone peaches, halved and pitted
½ red onion, minced
2 jalapeño peppers, cored, seeded, and minced
Juice of 1 lime
½ teaspoon ground cloves
½ teaspoon ground allspice
½ teaspoon coriander seeds, ground
½ cup light brown sugar, or to taste
¼ cup white wine vinegar
1 teaspoon salt, or to taste
Freshly ground black pepper to taste
Red pepper flakes to taste
¼ bunch fresh cilantro, chopped

Fresh Tomato Dressing

This is perfect over shrimp, drizzled onto avocados, or even used as a sauce for hot or cold chicken or fish. It tastes summery!

Purée all ingredients in the blender. Taste for salt and pepper. This dressing improves with age—try making it a day or two in advance.

Balsamic Vinegar

There are various types of Italian vinegar, but perhaps the most famous is blasamic vinegar. Balsamic vinegar is made from reduced wine and aged in special wood barrels for years. Each year's barrels are made of a different type of wood—the vinegar absorbs the flavor of the wood. Authentic balsamic vinegar ages for a minimum of 10 and up to 30 years.

Makes 2 cups, 16 servings

**Per Serving
(2 tablespoons)**

Calories: 78
GI: Very Low
Carbohydrates: 2 g.
Protein: 0 g.
Fat: 7 g.

1 pint cherry tomatoes
4 cloves roasted garlic
2 shallots
2 jalapeño peppers, cored and seeded
¼ cup stemmed, loosely packed fresh basil
¼ cup red wine or balsamic vinegar
½ cup extra-virgin olive oil
½ teaspoon celery salt
2 teaspoons Worcestershire sauce
Freshly ground black pepper to taste
½ teaspoon cayenne pepper, or to taste

Caramelized Onions

These are wonderful on everything from sandwiches to salads and as a garnish for roasts and stews.

Place the onions in a large sauté pan with the butter or olive oil. Over very low heat, sauté for 20 minutes, or until onions are browned but not burned.

Makes 1 cup

PER SERVING

Calories: 420
GI: Very Low
Carbohydrates: 75 g.
Protein: 9 g.
Fat: 12 g.

3 large Vidalia or other sweet onions, sliced ⅛-inch thick
1 tablespoon olive oil

Fruit Chutney with Pineapple, Pine Nuts, and Chilies

The combination of sweet and spicy is classic in Indian cuisine. This is lovely with chicken, rice, or fish.

Mix all ingredients in a bowl. Cover and refrigerate for 24 hours, stirring every few hours.

Makes 1-½ cups, 12 servings

PER SERVING (2 TABLESPOONS)

Calories: 37
GI: High
Carbohydrates: 6 g.
Protein: 1 g.
Fat: 1 g.

1 cup pineapple chunks, fresh
¼ cup pine nuts, toasted
2 green chilies, roasted, peeled, cored, and seeded
2 tablespoons brown sugar
1 teaspoon curry powder, or to taste
4 whole cloves
Juice of 1 lime
1 teaspoon salt
Freshly ground black pepper

Mustard-Curry Sauce for Seafood or Poultry

This is a wonderful summer sauce for shrimp, crabmeat, or cold chicken.

Makes 1 cup,
enough for 4 servings
of cold seafood salad

PER SERVING

Calories: 126
GI: Very Low
Carbohydrates: 4 g.
Protein: 0 g.
Fat: 13 g.

½ cup low-fat mayonnaise
½ cup low-fat sour cream
1 teaspoon curry powder
1 teaspoon Dijon-style mustard
½ teaspoon black pepper,
*   freshly ground*
1 tablespoon lemon juice,
*   fresh only*
Salt to taste
½ teaspoon onion powder
1 tablespoon fresh parsley

Place all ingredients in the blender and purée until smooth. Mix into seafood or chicken salad.

Varied Curries

Curry can refer to any kind of spiced, sauce-based dish that is usually eaten over rice. Curry is most often associated with Indian and Thai cooking and in the last few decades has become extremely popular in Britain.

Pomegranate Sauce

This is excellent with game or any kind of poultry.
Try it with grilled or roasted venison.

Mix all ingredients in a saucepan. Bring to a boil. Reduce heat and simmer until reduced to 1 cup. Its consistency should be syrupy.

Makes 1 cup, 8 servings

PER SERVING

Calories: 30
GI: Moderate
Carbohydrates: 11 g.
Protein: 0 g.
Fat: 0 g.

1-½ cups pomegranate juice
½ cup sugar substitute
Juice and rind of ½ orange, seeded
2 whole cloves

Cucumber, Dill, and Sour Cream

This recipe is marvelous with poached, chilled salmon. Use fresh herbs only!

Mix all ingredients in a bowl. Cover and refrigerate for 1 hour. Serve chilled.

Makes 2 cups, serves 4 as a sauce/dressing

PER SERVING

Calories: 62
GI: Very Low
Carbohydrates: 10 g.
Protein: 1 g.
Fat: 4 g.

1-½ cups cucumber, peeled and chopped
½ cup red onion, chopped fine
Juice of 1 lemon
1 teaspoon Tabasco sauce
½ cup low-fat sour cream
1 teaspoon celery salt, or to taste
½ cup fresh dill, finely minced
2 tablespoons minced chives
½ teaspoon sweet paprika, or to taste

Green Mayonnaise for Fish or Poultry

This is a classic served with cold salmon. Only fresh herbs will do! Dried herbs do not have the consistency, flavor, or color of fresh ones. This recipe "cooks" the eggs, but if you are worried about raw eggs, you can get pasteurized eggs.

Makes 1 cup, 8 servings

**PER SERVING
(2 TABLESPOONS)**

Calories: 183
GI: Zero
Carbohydrates: 0 g.
Protein: 1 g.
Fat: 21 g.

1 whole egg
1 egg yolk
Juice of ½ lemon
½ teaspoon Dijon-style
    mustard
¼ cup chives, chopped
¼ cup Italian flat-leaf parsley,
    chopped
1 tablespoon fresh thyme
    leaves
1 tablespoon fresh oregano
    leaves
½ teaspoon salt, or to taste
Freshly ground black pepper
    to taste
⅔ cup extra-virgin olive oil,
    warmed to 150°F

Place eggs, lemon juice, mustard, herbs, salt, and pepper in the blender. On low speed, very slowly add the olive oil, giving the eggs time to "digest" it. Chill and serve.

Italian Parsley versus Curly Parsley

Italian parsley, also known as flat leaf parsley, is easier to dice for recipes than the curly parsley you may be used to seeing. It also has a more pungent flavor than the somewhat bland taste of curly parsley. You can chew a bit of the extra parsley after a garlicky meal to ward off bad breath!

Mary Rose Sauce—Irish Mayonnaise

In Ireland, this is enormously popular as a dipping sauce for fish and chips.
It's also good with fried chicken and broiled fish.

Whisk all ingredients together and serve in an attractive cup or bowl.

1 cup, 8 servings

PER SERVING
(2 TABLESPOONS)

Calories: 80
GI: Very Low
Carbohydrates: 6 g.
Protein: 0 g.
Fat: 7 g.

6 ounces low-fat mayonnaise
1 ounce tomato paste
1 ounce malt vinegar
4 scallions, minced
2 tablespoons sweet red pepper,
*   roasted and minced*
½ teaspoon hot pepper sauce

Roasted Garlic

This is useful as a spread for bread and as an addition
to salad dressings and marinades.

1. Preheat oven to 350°F. Cut off top of garlic, ¼ inch down.

2. Make a pocket with aluminum foil and add garlic, olive oil, and water. Roast for 1 hour.

3. Separate individual cloves. Squeeze over bread, into dressings, or add to a variety of marinades.

Makes 1 head garlic

PER SERVING

Calories: 40
GI: Zero
Carbohydrates: 0 g.
Protein: 0 g.
Fat: 5 g.

1 head garlic
1 teaspoon olive oil
2 tablespoons water

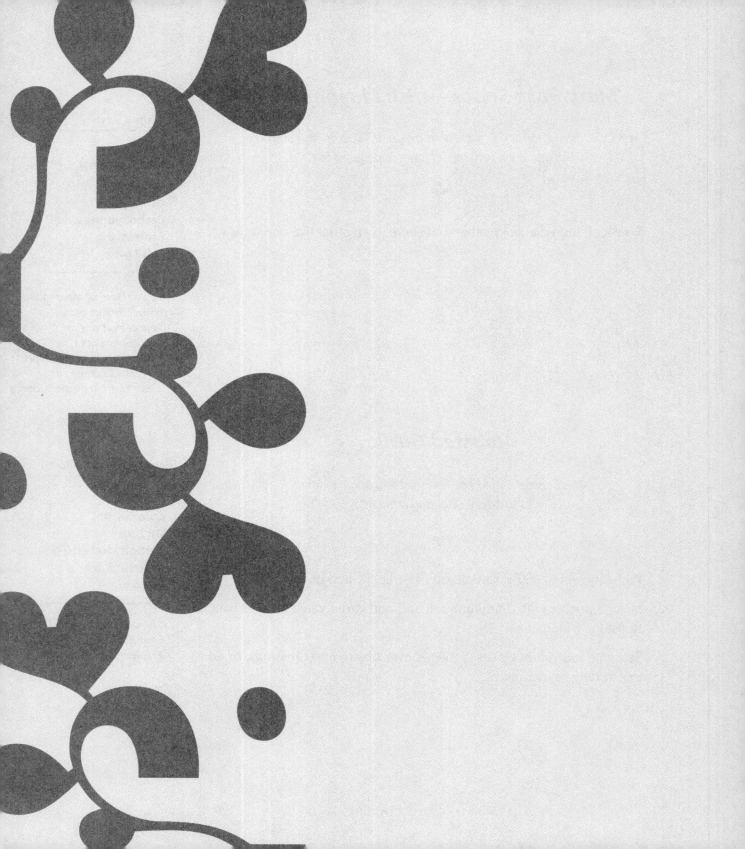

chapter 16
Desserts

Rice Pudding with Sour Cherries

*This recipe is wonderful for kids, giving them
long-lasting carbohydrates, fruit, and milk. Its creamy sweetness
blended with fall spices makes grown-ups love it, too!*

Serves 6

PER SERVING

Calories: 165
GI: Low
Carbohydrates: 26 g.
Protein: 6 g.
Fat: 5 g.

2 cups basmati rice, cooked
1-½ cups 2% milk
2 eggs
1 teaspoon vanilla
1 teaspoon salt
¼ cup sugar substitute
¼ teaspoon nutmeg
¼ teaspoon mace
*1 cup sour pie cherries,
    drained, not in sugar
    syrup*
1 tablespoon butter, soft
Nonstick spray

1. Preheat oven to 325°F. Spray a 2-quart baking dish with nonstick spray. Add the rice.

2. Whisk together the milk, eggs, vanilla, salt, sugar substitute, nutmeg, and mace. Stir in cherries and butter. Mix into the rice.

3. Bake for 50 minutes. Serve warm or chilled.

> *Substitute heart-healthy margarine for butter
> and replace 2% milk with nonfat milk.*

Sugar Substitutes

You can use a sugar substitute, such as Splenda, in almost any dessert recipe to lower your GI. The exceptions are in desserts that require caramelizing sugar. (These include flan and brittle.) Just follow directions but remember that substitutes are actually sweeter than sugar.

Whipped Cream

The best whipped cream does not come out of an aerosol can! Try making it yourself to create a rich, creamy topping for a variety of desserts.

Using an electric mixer or wire whisk (not a blender or food processor), beat the cream on medium low, adding the sugar substitute a bit at a time. Add vanilla. Don't overbeat, or you'll make butter!

1 cup whipped cream, 4 servings

PER SERVING

Calories: 90
GI: Very Low
Carbohydrates: 0 g.
Protein: 0 g.
Fat: 9 g.

½ cup whipping or heavy cream
1 teaspoon sugar substitute, or to taste
Optional: 1 teaspoon vanilla extract

Grilled Caramelized Pineapple

This is a perfect dessert that is quick and easy to make whenever you are grilling. You can get fresh pineapple, peeled, cored, and cut in fat circles.

1. Brush both sides of the pineapple slices with lime juice and sprinkle with brown sugar.

2. Place sugar-coated pineapple slices on a hot grill; turn after 3 minutes. Grill another 3 minutes.

3. When the pineapples are done, you should have a nice brown caramel color. Top with lemon sorbet and a drizzle of melted dark chocolate if you want to gild the lily.

Serves 4

PER SERVING

Calories: 29
GI: High
Carbohydrates: 13 g.
Protein: 1 g.
Fat: 0 g.

4 thick slices pineapple, about 1 inch each
Juice of ½ lime
4 teaspoons brown sugar

Old-Fashioned Apple and Peach Crisp

This is a perfect end-of-summer dish. The apples are just ripening, and the peaches are on their way out. Combining the two is wonderful! You can serve warm or chilled, plain, with whipped cream, or with ice cream!

Serves 4

PER SERVING

Calories: 360
GI: Moderate
Carbohydrates: 60 g.
Protein: 6 g.
Fat: 14 g.

2 tart apples, peeled, cored,
    and sliced
4 medium peaches, blanched,
    skins and pits removed,
    sliced
Juice of ½ lemon
½ cup flour
¼ cup dark brown sugar
½ teaspoon cinnamon
½ teaspoon salt
½ teaspoon coriander seed,
    ground
½ teaspoon cardamom seed,
    ground
1 cup oatmeal
½ stick butter, softened
Nonstick spray

1. Preheat the oven to 350°F. Prepare a gratin dish or baking dish with nonstick spray.

2. Distribute the apple and peach slices in the dish and sprinkle with lemon juice.

3. Using your hands, thoroughly mix together the flour, brown sugar, spices, oatmeal, and butter. Spread over the crisp and bake for 45 minutes, or until the fruit is bubbling and the top is brown. Serve with vanilla ice cream or whipped cream.

> *Substitute low-fat frozen yogurt for ice cream or whipped cream to make this a healthier dessert. You could also replace the butter with heart-healthy margarine.*

Baked Apples Stuffed with Nuts and Raisins

For breakfast or dessert, baked apples are a delightful, spicy, and warm treat.

Serves 2

Per Serving

Calories: 181
GI: Low
Carbohydrates: 28 g.
Protein: 1 g.
Fat: 8 g.

*2 large apples, such as
    Macintosh, Rome, or
    Granny Smith*
2 teaspoons brown sugar
½ teaspoon cinnamon
2 teaspoons chopped walnuts
2 teaspoons raisins
1 teaspoon butter

1. Preheat the oven to 350°F. Using a corer, remove the center portions of the apples, being careful not to cut through the bottom of the apple.

2. Form a cup with a double layer of aluminum foil, going ⅓ of the way up the apple. This will stabilize the apple when baking.

3. Mix together the brown sugar, cinnamon, walnuts, and raisins and stuff the mixture into the apples. Top each apple with 1 teaspoon of butter. Put 1 tablespoon of water into the aluminum foil cups.

4. Bake for 25 minutes, or until the apples are soft when pricked with a fork.

> ❤ *Replace butter with heart-healthy margarine.* ❤

Creamy Additions

The spices in these baked, stuffed apples and the tartness of the apples are both complemented nicely by dairy. You can serve these with a little cream poured over the top or a scoop of vanilla ice cream on the side for added richness.

Grilled Nectarines with Mascarpone and Raspberry Granité

Serves 2

PER SERVING

Calories: 108
GI: Low
Carbohydrates: 16 g.
Protein: 2 g.
Fat: 5 g.

2 nectarines, cut in halves,
  pits discarded
4 teaspoons mascarpone
  cheese
4 tablespoons raspberry
  granité (see page 255)
Optional: fresh raspberries
  for garnish

This is absolutely perfect for a summer night. The combination of mascarpone cheese, which is a rich, triple-cream cow's milk cheese, and the sweetness of the nectarines is sublime. Grilling the nectarines brings out their juicy flavor.

1. Place the nectarines, cut side down on a hot grill for 5 minutes.

2. Spoon the mascarpone into the depressions left by the pits. Add raspberry granité and serve immediately. If you like, top each nectarine half with a fresh raspberry.

Frosted Blueberries with Peach Ice

Serves 4

PER SERVING

Calories: 70
GI: Low
Carbohydrates: 24 g.
Protein: 1 g.
Fat: 0 g.

1 cup fresh blueberries
1 tablespoon confectioners'
  sugar
4 fresh peaches, blanched,
  halved, pitted, and skins
  removed
Juice of ½ lemon
½ cup sugar substitute
1-½ cups water

This is an icy treat on a hot day, and they are great at night, too!

1. Cover a baking sheet with aluminum foil. Rinse blueberries and place them while still damp on the sheet and freeze. After 2 hours, sprinkle with confectioners' sugar, roll to coat, cover with plastic wrap, and return to the freezer.

2. Place the peaches, lemon juice, sugar substitute, and water in the blender and purée until very smooth.

3. Pour the peach mixture into an ice cube tray and freeze for 2 hours. Remove and break up with a fork. Continue to freeze until you have a very grainy, icy mixture.

4. Fold the peach slush and blueberries together. Serve in wine goblets.

Raspberry Granité

*Nothing tastes fresher than the pure fruit ice in this recipe
and the following Spicy Apple Granité recipe.*

1. Bring all ingredients to a boil in a medium saucepan.

2. Reduce heat and simmer, covered for 10 minutes, or until the sugar substitute melts.

3. Force the mixture through a sieve and freeze, breaking up with a fork occasionally. Continue to freeze and break apart until you have a very grainy, icy mixture.

Champagne and Granité

Granité is a sweetened, often fruit-flavored ice with a granular texture. For this recipe, add a splash of champagne to the mixture before freezing to make an elegant dessert for entertaining.

Serves 4

PER SERVING

Calories: 61
GI: Low
Carbohydrates: 7 g.
Protein: 1 g.
Fat: 1 g.

1 quart raspberries
1 cup water
4 packets sugar substitute
1 tablespoon lemon juice
Pinch of salt

Makes 1 cup, 8 servings

PER SERVING

Calories: 126
GI: High
Carbohydrates: 21 g.
Protein: 1 g.
Fat: 5 g.

1 teaspoon unsalted butter
1 teaspoon Wondra quick-
    blending flour
1 ounce walnuts, chopped
1 ounce any mixed nuts,
    chopped
6 ounces maple syrup

Maple-Nut Sauce for Desserts

*This is rich, buttery, and delicious as a topping on
ice cream, pumpkin pie, and soufflé.*

Melt the butter in a saucepan. Stir in flour. Add nuts and sauté them. Stir in maple syrup and serve warm.

> ❤   *Substitute heart-healthy margarine for butter.*   ❤

Serves 4

PER SERVING

Calories: 79
GI: Low
Carbohydrates: 21 g.
Protein: 0 g.
Fat: 0 g.

4 Macintosh or other
    semisweet apples, peeled,
    cored, and quartered
1 packet sugar substitute, or
    to taste
1 teaspoon ground cinnamon
⅛ teaspoon ground nutmeg
⅛ teaspoon ground cloves
Juice and minced rind of ½
    lemon
¼ cup water, more depending
    on the juiciness of the
    apples
Pinch of salt

Spicy Apple Granité

*Try this as a topping for hot apple pie instead of ice cream, or just spoon it into
chilled martini glasses for an elegant and light dessert for entertaining.*

1. Mix all ingredients in a 1-quart saucepan. Bring to a boil; reduce heat to a simmer. Cover and cook for 10 minutes.

2. Allow mixture to cool for 30 minutes. Purée mixture in the blender and pour into an ice cube tray.

2. Freeze for 5 hours, breaking up with a fork every 2 hours. Serve when slushy and grainy.

Nut-Crusted Key Lime Pie

*Nut crusts are versatile and very good with almost any kind of pie,
and although nuts are fattening, they are still good for you—
containing high amounts of fiber and vitamin E.*

1. In the food processor or blender, mix the nuts, cracker crumbs, butter, brown sugar, and orange rind to the texture of oatmeal.

2. Prepare a 9" pie pan with nonstick spray and press the nut mixture into it. Bake in a 325°F oven for 30 minutes, or until crisp and lightly browned. Set aside to cool and then refrigerate.

3. In the blender, mix 1 cup of the water and all remaining ingredients but the egg whites and sugar substitute. Add the rest of the water and pour into a saucepan. Whisking constantly, bring to a boil. Cool until almost stiff.

4. Place the lime mixture in the well-chilled pie shell. Fold the sugar into the beaten egg whites and spread over lime filling.

5. Place pie under broiler set at 350°F until golden brown.

Serves 8

**Per Serving
(1-inch piece)**

Calories: 348
GI: Crust – Low; Filling – Zero
Carbohydrates: 68 g.
Protein: 6 g.
Fat: 27 g.

1 cup macadamia nuts, pecans, or walnuts, coarsely ground
1 cup graham cracker crumbs
1 stick butter, melted
1 tablespoon dark brown sugar
Rind of ½ orange
1-½ cups cold water
⅓ cup cornstarch
Juice of 3 limes
2 packets unflavored gelatin
2 tablespoons sugar substitute
2 egg yolks
3 egg whites, beaten stiff
Nonstick spray

Meringue Piecrust

Any number of fillings are wonderful in this piecrust.
It should be made the same day you use it. Once filled or
sitting out in a humid room, it will turn soggy.

1. Prepare a 9" pie pan with nonstick spray. Beat egg whites adding salt and then vinegar and sugar substitute. When stiff, fold in nuts.

2. Pile into pie pan. Bake at 175°F for 3 to 4 hours.

3. Let cool before filling.

Makes a 9″ piecrust

PER SERVING (8 SLICES)

Calories: 100
GI: Zero
Carbohydrates: 6 g.
Protein: 4 g.
Fat: 9 g.

4 egg whites
Pinch salt
1 teaspoon vinegar
½ cup sugar substitute, or to
    taste
½ cup toasted walnuts,
    hazelnuts, or pecans
Nonstick spray

Fruit and Cream Filling for Meringue Piecrust

This is the classic filling for Pavlova cake, a wonderful Australian dessert.
The cake is sometimes topped with peeled, sliced kiwi fruit in addition
to strawberries, which you could do for this recipe as well.

1. Using a cool meringue piecrust, slice the banana over the bottom of the crust.

2. Whip the cream with the sugar substitute and vanilla. Spoon and spread on half the whipped cream mixture.

3. Cover with the sliced strawberries; sprinkle with sugar substitute.

4. Cover with whipped cream and arrange the rest of the berries on top. Serve immediately.

Serves 8

PER SERVING
(CRUST NOT INCLUDED)

Calories: 116
GI: Very Low
Carbohydrates: 6g.
Protein: 0 g.
Fat: 9 g.

Meringue Piecrust (see above)
1 banana
1 cup heavy or whipping cream
2 teaspoons sugar substitute
1 teaspoon vanilla extract
1 pint strawberries, washed
    and hulled, half sliced, half
    left whole for top of pie
1 tablespoon sugar substitute

Raspberry or Strawberry Coulis

This is delectable over ice cream, sherbet, or sorbet.

Blend all ingredients in the blender. Strain and serve.

Makes 6 ounces, 6 servings

PER SERVING

Calories: 8
GI: Very Low
Carbohydrates: 2 g.
Protein: 0 g.
Fat: 0 g.

*8 ounces strawberries or
    raspberries, washed and
    hulled
1 teaspoon lemon juice
Sugar substitute to taste (start
    with one packet)*

Peach Coulis with Ginger

This can be frozen for future use.

Place the peaches in a saucepan with water. Boil for 2 to 3 minutes. Cool; remove pits and skins. Place in the blender with sugar substitute and lemon juice. Blend and serve.

Makes 1 cup, 4 servings

**PER SERVING
(2 OUNCES)**

Calories: 43
GI: Very Low
Carbohydrates: 11 g.
Protein: 1 g.
Fat: 0 g.

*4 medium-sized ripe peaches
½ cup water
1 teaspoon sugar substitute,
    or to taste
Juice of ½ lemon*

Strawberry Rhubarb Pudding

This is a wonderful flavor for spring. It's low-fat and low carb, as well as low GI.

Serves 4

PER SERVING

Calories: 195
GI: Very Low
Carbohydrates: 41 g.
Protein: 10 g.
Fat: 0 g.

1 envelope unflavored gelatin
¼ cup cold water
1 cup fresh rhubarb, cut in
    1-inch pieces
¼ cup water
½ pint strawberries, washed,
    hulled, and sliced (half
    reserved for topping)
½ cup Splenda sugar
    substitute for baking
2 cups nonfat vanilla yogurt

1. Place the gelatin and cold water in the jar of the blender.

2. In a saucepan, over medium heat, boil the rhubarb, water, and half the strawberries with the Splenda.

3. Add the hot fruit to the gelatin and pulse to chop and mix the gelatin with the fruit. Cool until room temperature.

4. Swirl the fruit and yogurt together and spoon into glasses or bowls. Add strawberries for topping.

Zabaglione

This Italian classic custard is an interactive dessert.
Made in a chafing dish, guests can take turns whisking until the
mixture foams up in a stunning show. You can serve this dish over sliced fruit,
such as strawberries, raspberries, or blueberries. If you do not have
a chafing dish, you can use a double boiler. The only drawback is that
it will not be spectacular for your guests to watch the egg foam!

Serves 6

PER SERVING

Calories: 143
GI: Zero
Carbohydrates: 10 g.
Protein: 3 g.
Fat: 5 g.

6 egg yolks
½ cup sugar substitute
⅔ cup Marsala wine

1. Set up the chafing dish but don't light the sterno or oil. Beat the egg yolks and sugar substitute together with an electric mixer until very pale, lemon yellow.

2. Whisk in the wine. Light the burner and place a pan of warm water in the base. Add egg mixture to the brazier pan.

3. Slowly heat the mixture, whisking constantly until it suddenly foams up and thickens slightly. Don't overcook, or you'll have Marsala-flavored scrambled eggs!

Make a Double Boiler

To make a double boiler, simmer about 1 inch of water in a deep saucepan. Sit a glass or metal bowl on the top of the saucepan. Take care that the simmering water does not touch the bottom of the bowl, or else you will scramble your eggs!

appendix A
Additional Information

http://www.diabetesnet.com
This Web site is useful for looking up information about the GI, as well as for determining the GI value of specific foods.

Irish Oatmeal
McCann's and Flavahan's are two brands of Irish oatmeal, which is cut more coarsely than quick oats for maximum advantage to low GI diets. These brands are available nationally in all major food chains.

Splenda, No Calorie Sweetener
This is an excellent sugar substitute for use in custards, pie fillings, cheesecakes, puddings, sweet sauces, frostings, homemade ice cream, and sorbets. It's not recommended when you want to brown a cookie or cake or caramelize a topping. Then, Splenda Sugar Blend for Baking is excellent—it has half the calories of sugar and provides enough sugar for texture and browning. Bakers like it because it holds up well—it doesn't break down or get bitter when exposed to heat.

Trader Joe's
A national chain, Trader Joe's has some of the most interesting foods available. Their frozen foods and other private label products are excellent, and their nuts are a bargain.

Wild Oats
Wild Oats is a chain of natural food stores specializing in organic fresh, frozen, dried, and prepared foods. They have many whole grain and low GI products from breads and cereals to cookies and cakes.

www.GlutenFreeMall.com
This is a fine source for all kinds of rice and a variety of flours. Whether you are worried about gluten or not, it's a resource for many products that may be hard to find in your local stores.

appendix B
Glycemic Index Reference Books

Brand-Miller, Jennie; Wolever, Thomas M.S.; Foster-Powell, Kaye; and Colagiuri, Stephen. *The Glucose Revolution Pocket Guide to Diabetes.* New York: Marlowe & Co., 2001.

Brand-Miller, Jennie; Wolever, Thomas M.S.; Foster-Powell, Kaye; and Colagiuri, Stephen. *The Glucose Revolution Pocket Guide to Sports Nutrition.* New York: Marlowe & Co., 2001.

Brand-Miller, Jennie; Wolever, Thomas M.S.; Foster-Powell, Kaye; and Colagiuri, Stephen. *The Glucose Revolution Pocket Guide to Your Heart.* New York: Marlowe & Co., 2001.

Brand-Miller, Jennie; Wolever, Thomas M.S.; Foster-Powell, Kaye; and Colagiuri, Stephen. *The New Glucose Revolution.* New York: Marlowe & Co., 1996, 2003.

Cunningham, Marion. *The Fannie Farmer Cookbook, 13th ed.* New York: Alfred Knopf, 1996.

Woodruff, Sandra. *The Good Carb Cookbook,* New York: Avery Press, 2001.

Index

The EVERYTHING Series!

BUSINESS & PERSONAL FINANCE

Everything® Budgeting Book
Everything® Business Planning Book
Everything® Coaching and Mentoring Book
Everything® Fundraising Book
Everything® Get Out of Debt Book
Everything® Grant Writing Book
Everything® Home-Based Business Book, 2nd Ed.
Everything® Homebuying Book, 2nd Ed.
Everything® Homeselling Book, 2nd Ed.
Everything® Investing Book, 2nd Ed.
Everything® Landlording Book
Everything® Leadership Book
Everything® Managing People Book
Everything® Negotiating Book
Everything® Online Business Book
Everything® Personal Finance Book
Everything® Personal Finance in Your 20s and 30s Book
Everything® Project Management Book
Everything® Real Estate Investing Book
Everything® Robert's Rules Book, $7.95
Everything® Selling Book
Everything® Start Your Own Business Book
Everything® Wills & Estate Planning Book

COMPUTERS

Everything® Online Auctions Book
Everything® Blogging Book

COOKING

Everything® Barbecue Cookbook
Everything® Bartender's Book, $9.95
Everything® Chinese Cookbook
Everything® Cocktail Parties and Drinks Book
Everything® College Cookbook
Everything® Cookbook
Everything® Cooking for Two Cookbook
Everything® Diabetes Cookbook
Everything® Easy Gourmet Cookbook
Everything® Fondue Cookbook
Everything® Gluten-Free Cookbook
Everything® Glycemic Index Cookbook
Everything® Grilling Cookbook

Everything® Healthy Meals in Minutes Cookbook
Everything® Holiday Cookbook
Everything® Indian Cookbook
Everything® Italian Cookbook
Everything® Low-Carb Cookbook
Everything® Low-Fat High-Flavor Cookbook
Everything® Low-Salt Cookbook
Everything® Meals for a Month Cookbook
Everything® Mediterranean Cookbook
Everything® Mexican Cookbook
Everything® One-Pot Cookbook
Everything® Pasta Cookbook
Everything® Quick Meals Cookbook
Everything® Slow Cooker Cookbook
Everything® Slow Cooking for a Crowd Cookbook
Everything® Soup Cookbook
Everything® Tex-Mex Cookbook
Everything® Thai Cookbook
Everything® Vegetarian Cookbook
Everything® Wild Game Cookbook
Everything® Wine Book, 2nd Ed.

CRAFT SERIES

Everything® Crafts—Baby Scrapbooking
Everything® Crafts—Bead Your Own Jewelry
Everything® Crafts—Create Your Own Greeting Cards
Everything® Crafts—Easy Projects
Everything® Crafts—Polymer Clay for Beginners
Everything® Crafts—Rubber Stamping Made Easy
Everything® Crafts—Wedding Decorations and Keepsakes

HEALTH

Everything® Alzheimer's Book
Everything® Diabetes Book
Everything® Health Guide to Adult Bipolar Disorder
Everything® Health Guide to Controlling Anxiety
Everything® Health Guide to Fibromyalgia
Everything® Hypnosis Book

Everything® Low Cholesterol Book
Everything® Massage Book
Everything® Menopause Book
Everything® Nutrition Book
Everything® Reflexology Book
Everything® Stress Management Book

HISTORY

Everything® American Government Book
Everything® American History Book
Everything® Civil War Book
Everything® Irish History & Heritage Book
Everything® Middle East Book

GAMES

Everything® 15-Minute Sudoku Book, $9.95
Everything® 30-Minute Sudoku Book, $9.95
Everything® Blackjack Strategy Book
Everything® Brain Strain Book, $9.95
Everything® Bridge Book
Everything® Card Games Book
Everything® Card Tricks Book, $9.95
Everything® Casino Gambling Book, 2nd Ed.
Everything® Chess Basics Book
Everything® Craps Strategy Book
Everything® Crossword and Puzzle Book
Everything® Crossword Challenge Book
Everything® Cryptograms Book, $9.95
Everything® Easy Crosswords Book
Everything® Easy Kakuro Book, $9.95
Everything® Games Book, 2nd Ed.
Everything® Giant Sudoku Book, $9.95
Everything® Kakuro Challenge Book, $9.95
Everything® Large-Print Crosswords Book
Everything® Lateral Thinking Puzzles Book, $9.95
Everything® Pencil Puzzles Book, $9.95
Everything® Poker Strategy Book
Everything® Pool & Billiards Book
Everything® Test Your IQ Book, $9.95
Everything® Texas Hold 'Em Book, $9.95
Everything® Travel Crosswords Book, $9.95
Everything® Word Games Challenge Book
Everything® Word Search Book

Bolded titles are new additions to the series.
All Everything® books are priced at $12.95 or $14.95, unless otherwise stated. Prices subject to change without notice.

HOBBIES

Everything® Candlemaking Book
Everything® Cartooning Book
Everything® Drawing Book
Everything® Family Tree Book, 2nd Ed.
Everything® Knitting Book
Everything® Knots Book
Everything® Photography Book
Everything® Quilting Book
Everything® Scrapbooking Book
Everything® Sewing Book
Everything® Woodworking Book

HOME IMPROVEMENT

Everything® Feng Shui Book
Everything® Feng Shui Decluttering Book, $9.95
Everything® Fix-It Book
Everything® Home Decorating Book
Everything® Homebuilding Book
Everything® Lawn Care Book
Everything® Organize Your Home Book

KIDS' BOOKS

All titles are $7.95
Everything® Kids' Animal Puzzle &
    Activity Book
Everything® Kids' Baseball Book, 4th Ed.
Everything® Kids' Bible Trivia Book
Everything® Kids' Bugs Book
Everything® Kids' Christmas Puzzle
    & Activity Book
Everything® Kids' Cookbook
Everything® Kids' Crazy Puzzles Book
Everything® Kids' Dinosaurs Book
**Everything® Kids' Gross Hidden Pictures
    Book**
Everything® Kids' Gross Jokes Book
Everything® Kids' Gross Mazes Book
Everything® Kids' Gross Puzzle and
    Activity Book
Everything® Kids' Halloween Puzzle
    & Activity Book
Everything® Kids' Hidden Pictures Book
Everything® Kids' Horses Book
Everything® Kids' Joke Book
Everything® Kids' Knock Knock Book
Everything® Kids' Math Puzzles Book
Everything® Kids' Mazes Book
Everything® Kids' Money Book
Everything® Kids' Nature Book

**Everything® Kids' Pirates Puzzle and
    Activity Book**
Everything® Kids' Puzzle Book
Everything® Kids' Riddles & Brain Teasers Book
Everything® Kids' Science Experiments Book
Everything® Kids' Sharks Book
Everything® Kids' Soccer Book
Everything® Kids' Travel Activity Book

KIDS' STORY BOOKS

Everything® Fairy Tales Book

LANGUAGE

Everything® Conversational Japanese Book
    (with CD), $19.95
Everything® French Grammar Book
Everything® French Phrase Book, $9.95
Everything® French Verb Book, $9.95
**Everything® German Practice Book with
    CD, $19.95**
Everything® Inglés Book
Everything® Learning French Book
Everything® Learning German Book
Everything® Learning Italian Book
Everything® Learning Latin Book
Everything® Learning Spanish Book
Everything® Sign Language Book
Everything® Spanish Grammar Book
Everything® Spanish Phrase Book, $9.95
Everything® Spanish Practice Book
    (with CD), $19.95
Everything® Spanish Verb Book, $9.95

MUSIC

Everything® Drums Book (with CD), $19.95
Everything® Guitar Book
**Everything® Guitar Chords Book with CD,
    $19.95**
Everything® Home Recording Book
Everything® Playing Piano and Keyboards
    Book
Everything® Reading Music Book (with CD),
    $19.95
Everything® Rock & Blues Guitar Book
    (with CD), $19.95
Everything® Songwriting Book

NEW AGE

Everything® Astrology Book, 2nd Ed.
Everything® Dreams Book, 2nd Ed.
Everything® Love Signs Book, $9.95

Everything® Numerology Book
Everything® Paganism Book
Everything® Palmistry Book
Everything® Psychic Book
Everything® Reiki Book
Everything® Tarot Book
Everything® Wicca and Witchcraft Book

PARENTING

Everything® Baby Names Book, 2nd Ed.
Everything® Baby Shower Book
Everything® Baby's First Food Book
Everything® Baby's First Year Book
Everything® Birthing Book
Everything® Breastfeeding Book
Everything® Father-to-Be Book
Everything® Father's First Year Book
Everything® Get Ready for Baby Book
Everything® Get Your Baby to Sleep Book,
    $9.95
Everything® Getting Pregnant Book
Everything® Homeschooling Book
Everything® Mother's First Year Book
Everything® Parent's Guide to Children
    and Divorce
Everything® Parent's Guide to Children
    with ADD/ADHD
Everything® Parent's Guide to Children
    with Asperger's Syndrome
Everything® Parent's Guide to Children
    with Autism
Everything® Parent's Guide to Children with
    Bipolar Disorder
Everything® Parent's Guide to Children
    with Dyslexia
Everything® Parent's Guide to Positive
    Discipline
Everything® Parent's Guide to Raising a
    Successful Child
**Everything® Parent's Guide to Raising
    Boys**
**Everything® Parent's Guide to Raising
    Siblings**
Everything® Parent's Guide to Tantrums
Everything® Parent's Guide to the Overweight
    Child
Everything® Parent's Guide to the Strong-
    Willed Child
Everything® Parenting a Teenager Book
Everything® Potty Training Book, $9.95
Everything® Pregnancy Book, 2nd Ed.

Bolded titles are new additions to the series.
All Everything® books are priced at $12.95 or $14.95, unless otherwise stated. Prices subject to change without notice.

Everything® Pregnancy Fitness Book
Everything® Pregnancy Nutrition Book
Everything® Pregnancy Organizer, $15.00
Everything® Toddler Book
Everything® Toddler Activities Book
Everything® Tween Book
Everything® Twins, Triplets, and More Book

PETS

Everything® Boxer Book
Everything® Cat Book, 2nd Ed.
Everything® Chihuahua Book
Everything® Dachshund Book
Everything® Dog Book
Everything® Dog Health Book
Everything® Dog Training and Tricks Book
Everything® German Shepherd Book
Everything® Golden Retriever Book
Everything® Horse Book
Everything® Horse Care Book
Everything® Horseback Riding Book
Everything® Labrador Retriever Book
Everything® Poodle Book
Everything® Pug Book
Everything® Puppy Book
Everything® Rottweiler Book
Everything® Small Dogs Book
Everything® Tropical Fish Book
Everything® Yorkshire Terrier Book

REFERENCE

Everything® Car Care Book
Everything® Classical Mythology Book
Everything® Computer Book
Everything® Divorce Book
Everything® Einstein Book
Everything® Etiquette Book, 2nd Ed.
Everything® Inventions and Patents Book
Everything® Mafia Book
Everything® Mary Magdalene Book
Everything® Philosophy Book
Everything® Psychology Book
Everything® Shakespeare Book

RELIGION

Everything® Angels Book
Everything® Bible Book
Everything® Buddhism Book
Everything® Catholicism Book

Everything® Christianity Book
Everything® Freemasons Book
Everything® History of the Bible Book
Everything® Jewish History & Heritage Book
Everything® Judaism Book
Everything® Kabbalah Book
Everything® Koran Book
Everything® Prayer Book
Everything® Saints Book
Everything® Torah Book
Everything® Understanding Islam Book
Everything® World's Religions Book
Everything® Zen Book

SCHOOL & CAREERS

Everything® Alternative Careers Book
Everything® College Major Test Book
Everything® College Survival Book, 2nd Ed.
Everything® Cover Letter Book, 2nd Ed.
Everything® Get-a-Job Book
Everything® Guide to Being a Paralegal
Everything® Guide to Being a Real Estate Agent
Everything® Guide to Starting and Running a Restaurant
Everything® Job Interview Book
Everything® New Nurse Book
Everything® New Teacher Book
Everything® Paying for College Book
Everything® Practice Interview Book
Everything® Resume Book, 2nd Ed.
Everything® Study Book
Everything® Teacher's Organizer, $16.95

SELF-HELP

Everything® Dating Book, 2nd Ed.
Everything® Great Sex Book
Everything® Kama Sutra Book
Everything® Self-Esteem Book

SPORTS & FITNESS

Everything® Fishing Book
Everything® Golf Instruction Book
Everything® Pilates Book
Everything® Running Book
Everything® Total Fitness Book
Everything® Weight Training Book
Everything® Yoga Book

TRAVEL

Everything® Family Guide to Hawaii
Everything® Family Guide to Las Vegas, 2nd Ed.
Everything® Family Guide to New York City, 2nd Ed.
Everything® Family Guide to RV Travel & Campgrounds
Everything® Family Guide to the Walt Disney World Resort®, Universal Studios®, and Greater Orlando, 4th Ed.
Everything® Family Guide to Cruise Vacations
Everything® Family Guide to the Caribbean
Everything® Family Guide to Washington D.C., 2nd Ed.
Everything® Guide to New England
Everything® Travel Guide to the Disneyland Resort®, California Adventure®, Universal Studios®, and the Anaheim Area

WEDDINGS

Everything® Bachelorette Party Book, $9.95
Everything® Bridesmaid Book, $9.95
Everything® Elopement Book, $9.95
Everything® Father of the Bride Book, $9.95
Everything® Groom Book, $9.95
Everything® Mother of the Bride Book, $9.95
Everything® Outdoor Wedding Book
Everything® Wedding Book, 3rd Ed.
Everything® Wedding Checklist, $9.95
Everything® Wedding Etiquette Book, $9.95
Everything® Wedding Organizer, $15.00
Everything® Wedding Shower Book, $9.95
Everything® Wedding Vows Book, $9.95
Everything® Weddings on a Budget Book, $9.95

WRITING

Everything® Creative Writing Book
Everything® Get Published Book, 2nd Ed.
Everything® Grammar and Style Book
Everything® Guide to Writing a Book Proposal
Everything® Guide to Writing a Novel
Everything® Guide to Writing Children's Books
Everything® Guide to Writing Research Papers
Everything® Screenwriting Book
Everything® Writing Poetry Book
Everything® Writing Well Book

Available wherever books are sold!
To order, call 800-289-0963, or visit us at *www.everything.com*
Everything® and everything.com® are registered trademarks of F+W Publications, Inc.